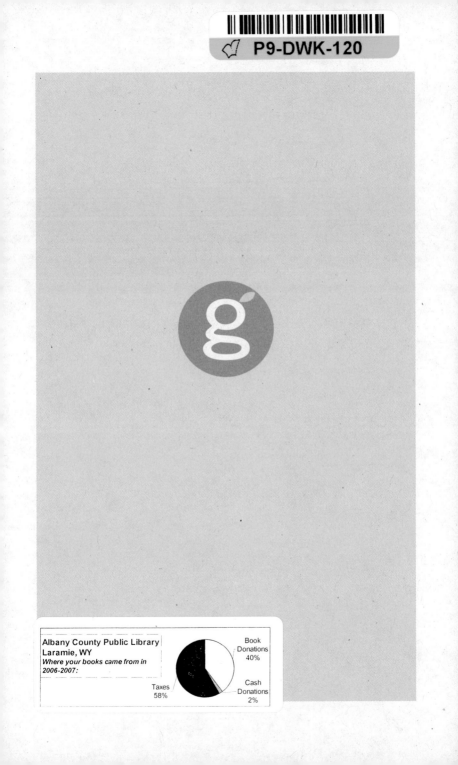

the green book

The EVERYDAY GUIDE to SAVING THE PLANET
ONE SIMPLE STEP at a TIME

ELIZABETH ROGERS and **THOMAS M. KOSTIGEN**

with a Foreword by
Cameron Diaz and William McDonough

Three Rivers Press
New York

Published in the United States by Three Rivers Press, an imprint of the
Crown Publishing Group, a division of Random House, Inc., New York.
www.crownpublishing.com

Three Rivers Press and the Tugboat design are registered trademarks
of Random House, Inc.

Library of Congress Cataloging-in-Publication Data

Rogers, Elizabeth (Elizabeth Kendall), 1965–
The green book : the everyday guide to saving the planet one simple step at
a time / Elizabeth Rogers and Thomas M. Kostigen ; with a foreword by
Cameron Diaz and William McDonough.
        p. cm.
Includes bibliographical references.
1. Environmental protection—Citizen participation. 2. Environmentalism.
        I. Kostigen, Thomas. II. Title.
TD171.7.R64 2007
333.72—dc22   2007013222

ISBN 978-0-307-38135-4

Printed in the United States of America

10 9

First Edition

For Emmett

contents

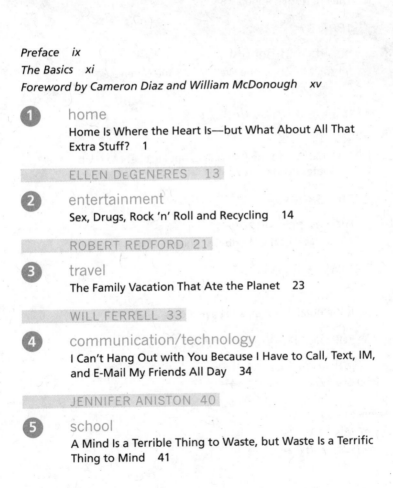

preface

Like three-year-olds, we kept asking the question "Why?" Why should we really turn off the lights in our homes? Why should we recycle? Why should we, as environmentally conscious freaks of the universe, really care about any of the things we are told make a difference? Why are we given dry, obtuse information from environmentalists who don't take into account the reality of our daily lives? Why are diapers poised to destroy the world?

There had to be some answers for the simple things. We searched the Internet for a connection—between what we do and what that action does: tying together our use of chopsticks to the deforestation and back to the price of our takeout, and so on. But we couldn't find many answers to our questions about what difference an individual action makes—at least none that really hit home.

When we trudge our garbage cans to the sidewalk every week—the blue for recyclables, the green for yard trash, the black for garbage—and we see our neighbors doing the same, we realize that we are all good citizens out of habit. But what would happen if we took it a step further and gave people new choices and explanations for what they do: why divvying up their waste makes a difference to the world?

Not since that famous 1970s TV commercial of a Native American crying at the sight of trash by the side of the road has there been a message or a campaign that speaks to cause and effect yet is easily understandable. That's why we created **The Green Book**. It looks at things differently, from a very basic point of view: what we do and what that does. And it answers all the questions we could come up with as to why what we do matters to the planet.

What we didn't want to do is create another deadly triple-D book—dull, dry, and dense. Instead, we strove to create solutions that are easy to understand and accessible. Neither of us lives in a tree or rides a stationary bicycle in a closet to generate electricity for our homes. We bet you don't, either.

This book is derived from our desire to be environmentally friendly while remaining selfish consumers. We think people have been waiting for this type of perspective. So here, in one place, are lots of answers to the question "Why?"

the basics

While **The Green Book** is a starting point for anyone who wants to become more environmentally friendly, there are some basic terms and terminology that may need to be explained. We broke down the book's solutions to explain how waste, water, energy, and time can be saved. These are the big areas we focused on because they involve so many issues. And saving each has a measurable positive impact on our planet.

Here are a few definitions and explanations of important items you'll hear about throughout **The Green Book.**

kilowatt-hours

These are units of energy typically found on your utility bill that tell you how much power you are using—and, of course, how much it's costing you to use that power. Usually, kWh are used to measure electrical power or natural gas use.

This is important because: Coal is what's used most to create electrical power. Coal is burned to make steam to power generators that make electricity. So, the more kWh you use, the more likely coal is burned (although some utilities use water or wind or other sources to generate power). Burning coal is a big source of harmful pollution and carbon emissions that can lead to global warming.

landfills

A landfill is a nice way of saying a dump or a trash site.

This is important because: Landfills not only take up land space that could be left natural or used for other purposes, but they can lead to air and water pollution issues in the local environment.

e-waste

Electronic waste consists of any discarded electronic appliance.

This is important because: Electronic appliances contain parts made from hazardous materials and need special care when they're disposed of. Otherwise those chemicals can leak into groundwater or get incinerated and create toxic air pollution.

recycling

Recycling prevents materials from being wasted by reprocessing them into new products. Recycled materials are usually "preconsumer" recycled products that are made out of scraps and trimmings. Postconsumer recycled materials are made out of things that have been used and reprocessed.

This is important because: Recycling prevents the need for more raw materials to be used when making things; therefore it saves natural resources. Recycling also helps save energy because it reduces the need to manufacture new things.

renewable resources

Renewable resources are those natural resources that regenerate, such as wind, water, trees, and sunlight.

This is important because: Renewable resources are never in danger of running out for good, only of our using more of their supply at a rate faster than they can regenerate.

nonrenewable resources

Nonrenewable resources are those things we use that are of more limited supply, such as oil, natural gas, and coal.

This is important because: Nonrenewable resources aren't sustainable, which means there is a danger we could run out of them and we'd have to seek out alternative replacements or solutions.

plastic

Plastic comes in many different forms and is made largely from synthetic material. And this material is composed mostly of petroleum.

This is important because: Some plastics, such as a common type called polyvinyl chloride, or PVC, can be worse for the environment than others because they're made from more toxic materials. So when these types of plastic are disposed of, they can release toxic fumes if burned or pollute the ground and water when they are buried in landfills.

pollution

Pollution is when harmful substances are released into the environment.

This is important because: Pollution can infect the water, air, and ground. Pollutants can cause diseases and illnesses and even kill us.

global warming

Global warming, sometimes called climate change, is when the earth's average temperature begins to rise.

This is important because: Global warming can cause sea levels to rise, intensify storms and weather patterns, and increase the likelihood that diseases will spread faster and farther around the planet.

waste

Waste is all our unwanted material: rubbish, trash, garbage, or junk.

This is important because: Some waste can be recovered and recycled.

Other types of waste are biodegradable, which means they "naturally" degrade into the earth. But some types of waste continue to pile up, so much so that the earth could be completely covered in it if we don't manage waste properly.

water

Only 3 percent of the water on earth is freshwater; the rest is saltwater.

This is important because: Fresh drinking water supplies are becoming increasingly scarce. Only 20 percent of the world's population has running water, and more than one billion people do not have any access to clean water.

paper

Paper is made mostly from wood pulp, which is made from trees, and water.

This is important because: Paper is the most common form of waste. Much of it can be recycled, but that still means more energy has to be used to reprocess it. Using less paper means saving energy, trees, water, and the chemicals needed in the manufacturing process. Trees are important because they prevent erosion and they absorb carbon from the air and turn it into the oxygen we breathe.

foreword

On a warm and breezy day in Los Angeles, award-winning architect William McDonough, a *Time* magazine "Hero for the Planet," visited Cameron Diaz's home to talk about this book, their individual "green" awakenings, and their common outlook on the world.

William McDonough: I was born in Tokyo. And I remember lying on my back on a futon at two o'clock in the morning in a Japanese house with paper walls, listening to the fountains and the *koi* out there. Listening, you could hear what they called the honey wagons come and collect all the sewage from the latrines and then go off to the farms in the middle of the night. You'd hear the whole city rumbling with carts taking out the sewage. Then in the morning you'd hear all the carts coming back in with tofu. That's what you'd have for breakfast, tofu. So you would remember, "Out went the waste, in came the food." I thought that's the way the world worked: that out went the waste and in came the food.

Then I went to Hong Kong. In a way, I lived in the future because I lived in a place with six million people on four hundred square miles. When we look at what cities in the middle of this century are going to be like, they will be located on large bodies of water, and the crowding will be amazing. Eighty percent of the world's population and 80 percent of the world's cities will be megacities like this. Hong Kong was the future megacity. There, people were dying of all sorts of diseases and starvation. It was terrible. This was just after the Communists took over in China, and all the refugees had gone to Hong Kong. We had four hours of water every fourth day. So the idea that you would save water is not unnatural to me. To brush your teeth, you would use a glass that you had saved water in for three days.

I had a whole childhood of this, things like that. My grandparents lived in a log cabin on the Puget Sound and raised oysters, composted, and recycled aluminum foil and put away vegetables for the winter. Then I went to Westport, Connecticut, for public high school, and it was all American stuff. It blew my mind. The guys left the showers running in the gym—hot water—and just walked right out. They didn't care. They just went out and hopped in their cars and roared away. I've never seen so much waste in my whole life. It made me an outcast because I was in high school and I'd be running around turning off the water. They thought I was a bit odd.

Then when I was at Yale—I started Yale for graduate school in 1973 as an architecture student—we had the first oil crisis. So all of sudden it was sort of like, "Wait a minute, we've got to deal with this now."

Cameron Diaz: My grandmother raised her own livestock in her backyard, her own vegetables in her backyard. And it was just here in the Valley next to Glendale, next to where the California Pizza Kitchen is right now. It was a different era and a different mentality. She raised her first four children there.

I watched my grandmother reuse tinfoil and plastic bags. And when she was finished with a loaf of bread, she kept that plastic bag and she would use it for something. She would make soap out of the fat drippings off of the meat she cooked. Nothing went to waste. Everything was reused and recycled. So I had that as an example.

I don't think that example exists for the generation right now. My grandmother lived a true sustainable existence. Everything she took from the land, she put back. Everything that she put back, she would take out again. It was a continuous cycle. And I witnessed that, and I was influenced a lot by that. My mother was influenced by that, and she passed it on to me. We need to be the examples now.

I never got into the environmental movement [before] because I really didn't connect to what was being said and how it was being said. I'm a selfish American. I don't want to give it all up. But at the same time, I found that I was already practicing the basics, everything from recycling to composting to saving energy to hybrid cars. I had been pursuing those things myself without knowing that they were part of the movement. Then I started listening more closely to what was being said because I was looking for a way in. I wanted to do more than what I was doing just for myself. I wanted to help other people do more.

What grabbed me about Bill is that he is a creative person. It isn't like his ideas are so far out that you can't grasp them. They all made perfect sense to me. And it was being said in a way that you don't want to be less bad. You don't want to be slapped on the back of the hand. You want to be productive. And that's how you get things done. That's what makes people respond. It isn't about cutting everything out. It is about creating something better. And that's something that I think is inspiring and something that brought me into the environmental movement. Nobody has all the answers right now. Yet every day we get closer to another answer. It may not be the answer to everything, 'cause that doesn't come. There is no one thing that we can all do that will make it all better. It's about making the best choices that are available.

Look at how long it's taken us to create what we have today and all we've done efficiency-wise, product-wise, and quality-wise—all of the things that we as Americans gain comfort in and expect to have available to us. We're doing pretty well. We're in a good place. It's an exciting time to be alive. We can figure out how to maintain our lifestyles and the health of the planet if we do it right. And that's what I want. I don't want to be running around barefoot, pushing my car like Barney Rubble. I don't want to go back to the Stone Age. I just want to maintain what we have for a long period of time—forever. How nice would that be? I'm very selfish.

William McDonough: The world often sees environmentalism or being green as being less bad. It's really not about being less bad, it's about being more good. So I think that's the difference. When all of a sudden you realize that we have to become a creative force, not just a less destructive force. That's a big revelation.

Cameron Diaz: It's a huge revelation. And that is what is so inspiring.

I really think of it as just the way things should be, the natural order of things. It's not about us. We were a successful society before we started building things and using up resources the way we do now. Human beings existed on this planet in harmony and in balance with it. There was a give and take between us and our resources. Now all of a sudden we feel like everything is getting kicked out from underneath us. It's imperative for us to pay attention to what our resources are doing, what we are doing to our resources, and how we are existing on this planet.

If you think of it as taking away something, withholding something, and not having everything that we want, then nobody wants to participate in that. Nobody wants to be a part of it. But the idea of still getting everything that we want, but just doing it in the right way, in a good way—like you said, not less bad but more good—that is the real goal.

William McDonough: This is about sharing and having enough to share. It should be a celebration of abundance, instead of anxieties about limits. I think that's really important. In our book *Cradle to Cradle: Remaking the Way We Make Things,* Michael Braungart and I are not looking at the world and saying, "Oh no, we are running out of everything!" We are looking at it and saying if we are able to recharacterize all the things that we made into perpetual clean products, then we could celebrate the abundance of this material rather than being terrified about what we are going to do if it's diluted.

Cameron Diaz: How do we move into that? To me, that's the creative part.

William McDonough: I think that's one of the important things about this book. It doesn't just say, "Turn off your light bulbs." Or, "You don't need a message machine if you can use voice mail." It's not going to be go without, go without, or cut back, cut back, whatever. The tone is more like, "Isn't it marvelous that voice mail happens to work really well and it's there all the time and therefore another appliance has hit the dust." That's an interesting way to look at it rather than saying people should not buy anything shrill. We ought to do a global search for the word *should* and the word *must* and put in *can* and *could*. You *can* do this. Not you *must* do this. You *can*, that is the creative act. *Must* is an instruction. *Can* is an openness to creativity. So we ought to decide what we *can* do.

Cameron Diaz: It's exciting to have a book like this where you can flip through and go see what you can do, what you can do instead of what you should have done. And be able to look at it and say, "Okay, there's an option, that's a thing that I can work toward changing my habits of doing on a day-to-day basis." Or even on a one-off, like buying a new pair of sneakers: "I'll have these sneakers forever now that my foot stopped growing. Someday we could find a perfect green shoe. But my best choice now is the ones with the recycled soles. . . ."

home

Home Is Where the Heart Is—but What About All That Extra Stuff?

THE BIG PICTURE

There are about 1.6 billion homes in the world, about 100 million in the United States alone. Yours is where you spend most of your time. It's where you use the most energy and water and create the most amount of waste.

On average, you create 4.5 pounds of trash every day. Over the course of your life, that will total six hundred times your average adult weight . . . in garbage. Broken down, your torso would be paper. One leg would be yard trimmings, the other food scraps. One arm would be plastic with a rubber hand. The other would be metal with a wood hand. Your head would be glass, and your neck would be all the other stuff. In the end, we will each leave a ninety-thousand-pound legacy of trash for our grandchildren.

But waste isn't our biggest impact on the planet: Americans use at least twice as much water and energy per person as anyone else in the world. Those are big problems considering there's a scarcity of both to go around.

By 2025, the world must increase its water supply by 22 percent in order to meet its needs. Meanwhile, 40 percent of the drinking water supplied to homes is flushed down the toilet.

As far as energy in the home goes, it's used mostly for heating and cooling.

Keeping all this in mind, we've created the "Simple Steps" to be just that. Taking into account all the points of the Big Picture, they allow you to make the biggest positive planetary impact with the least amount of effort.

The Simple Steps

1. **Take a shorter shower.** Every two minutes you save on your shower can conserve more than ten gallons of water. And that can add up: If everyone in the country saved just one gallon from their daily shower, over the course of a year it would equal twice the amount of freshwater withdrawn from the Great Lakes every day. The Great Lakes are the world's largest source of freshwater.

2. **Set your thermostat a degree higher for air-conditioning and a degree lower for heating,** and you could save $100 per year on your utility bill. Keep adjusting and you'll save even more. If every home in America turned the dial, we could save more than $10 billion per year on energy costs, enough to provide a year's worth of gasoline, electricity, and natural gas to every person in Iowa.

3. **Recycle.** If everyone in America simply separated the paper, plastic, glass, and aluminum products from the trash and tossed them into a recycling bin, we could decrease the amount of waste sent to landfills by 75 percent. Currently, it takes an area the size of Pennsylvania to dump all our waste each year.

THE LITTLE THINGS

In the Kitchen

Composting

Keep your kitchen scraps from fruits, vegetables, and coffee grounds in a composting bin or container. Try adding them to your garden or starting a compost site in the yard. You'll grow a better garden, create deeper topsoil, recycle nutrients, and save landfill space. If, over the course of a year, everyone in the United States composted their kitchen scraps instead of sending them away with the trash, the organic waste diverted from landfills could make a three-foot-high compost pile to cover the city of San Francisco.

Dishwasher

Run full loads in your dishwasher and save energy, and don't pre-rinse your dishes before putting them in. Do both and you'll save up to 20 gallons of water per dish load, or 7,300 gallons over a year. That's as much water as the average person drinks in a lifetime. (If you must handwash, turn off the tap while you scrub.)

Food Waste

When cooking and baking, try to avoid wasting food by using perishable ingredients before they spoil, measuring carefully, and saving leftovers for future meals instead of throwing them away. If you could reduce the amount of food wasted in your household by just twenty-five grams per day (about the weight of a slice of bread), you'd save twenty pounds of food annually—roughly enough to make sixteen meals. If all U.S. households reduced their food waste by this amount, the savings would be enough to provide three meals per day for a whole year to each of the 1.35 million children in the United States who are homeless.

Garbage Disposal

Use cold water when you run your garbage disposal. Better yet, try not to use it at all by composting your food waste or disposing of it in the trash. Your drain will be less clogged, and you'll save money on maintaining your septic system. Disposal waste can disrupt nutrient balances in water and soil ecosystems, which in turn can harm wildlife.

Microwave

Keep your microwave clean and you'll be able to maximize its energy. This means less electricity used, less money spent, and less time cooking. Microwaves are between 3.5 and 4.8 times more energy efficient than traditional electric ovens. If it costs ten cents to cook one item in a microwave, it would cost forty-eight cents to cook the same item in a standard oven. If everyone in North America cooked exclusively with a microwave for a year, we'd save as much energy as the entire continent of Africa consumes during that same time.

Preheating

If you're broiling, roasting, or baking a dish that will cook for an hour or more, don't bother preheating your oven. Even for breads and cakes, never preheat for longer than ten minutes. If you reduce the amount of time your oven is on by one hour per year, you'll save an average of two kilowatt-hours of energy. If 30 percent of U.S. households could each reduce total oven preheating time by just one hour per year, the sixty million kilowatt-hours of energy saved could bake a dozen cookies for every American.

Refrigerator

Keep your head out of the refrigerator and the door closed! The refrigerator is the single biggest energy-consuming kitchen appliance, and opening the refrigerator door accounts for between $30 and $60 of a typical family's electricity bill each year. The amount of energy saved in a year by more efficient refrigerator usage could be enough to light every house in the United States for more than four and a half months straight.

Storage Containers

Instead of using plastic, store your food in glass or porcelain containers. Fewer chemicals will likely leach from the container into the food. Chemicals that transfer from plastic to food and from food to body may cause health risks.

Stove

Use the right-size pot on your stove burners. You could save about $36 annually for an electric range or $18 for a gas range. Five percent of the energy bought and used per person in the United States is for preparing and cooking food. Over a year, this exceeds twice the energy a person in Africa uses to power everything in his or her life.

Trash Bags

Use leftover paper or plastic bags as liners for your trash cans. You'll save money and time shopping in the trash-liner bag aisle. The average cost of twenty kitchen trash bags is $5. When one ton of plastic bags is reused, the energy equivalent of eleven barrels of oil is saved. When one ton of paper bags is reused, up to seventeen trees are spared.

Water Filters

If you want to be sure the tap water in your house is clean, try installing water filters on your faucets instead of buying bottled water—you'll save money over time and get better-tasting water. You can buy a water filter for as little as $29, or about a month's worth of bottled water (if you drink a liter a day). About 1.5 million tons of plastic are used in the bottling of 89 billion liters of drinking water each year. That's enough plastic to make two water filters for every household on the planet. One billion people around the world lack access to clean drinking water.

In the Bathroom

Brushing Your Teeth

Turn off the tap while you brush your teeth. You'll conserve up to 5 gallons of water per day. Throughout the entire United States, the daily savings could add up to 1.5 billion gallons—more water than is consumed per day across all of New York City.

Shaving

Instead of letting the water run when you brush your teeth, brush while you're waiting for the water to get hot for your shave. You could save time and money on water, up to 1,825 gallons of water per "brushaver" each year. This much water would fill your bathtub more than thirty-five times!

Shower Curtains

Avoid using plastic liners (you don't really need them) with your shower curtains, and you'll keep unnatural vinyl plastics out of landfills. PVC plastic waste amounts to 1.23 million tons per year, and none of it is recyclable.

Toilet

Try to flush just one less time per day, and you'll save about 4.5 gallons of water—as much water as the average person in Africa uses for a whole day of drinking, cooking, bathing, and cleaning.

Tub

Plug the drain in the tub before turning on the water when you take a bath. You'll save time and money. The average bathtub faucet flows between three and five gallons of water per minute. Just one less gallon of water used per person in the United States per day can add up to more

than one hundred billion gallons per year. This amount is
the volume of rainwater that falls each week on Lloró, Colombia
wettest place on earth.

In the Living Room

Fireplace

Keep your fireplace damper closed unless a fire is going. An open damper can let 8 percent of the heat in your home escape. In the summer, cool air escapes. That can add up to about $100 a year—up the chimney.

Junk Mail

Rid yourself of junk mail—or at least recycle it. The average U.S. household receives 1.5 trees' worth of junk mail each year, and many of these trees are thrown right into the trash. If you want to reduce the amount of junk mail you receive, you'll need to register with the Mail Preference Service. It costs a buck, but you can do it easily online at www.dmaconsumers.org/cgi/offmailinglist. For the junk mail you continue to receive, remember to toss it in the recycling bin instead of throwing it out with the garbage. You can even recycle plastic window envelopes. If all Americans recycled their junk mail, $370 million in landfill dumping fees could be saved each year.

Light Bulbs

Dust your light bulbs and change them—to compact fluorescent—only when they burn out. You'll increase energy efficiency and light output, and because electricity production generates pollution, you'll also help promote cleaner air. If every American home changed out just five regular light fixtures or the bulbs in them with more energy-efficient compact fluorescent ones, we'd keep more than one trillion pounds of greenhouse gases out of our air—equal to the emissions of eight million cars. That's $6 billion in energy savings for Americans.

Matches vs. Lighters

When choosing between matches and lighters, choose matches. For lighters, both the plastic casing and the butane fuel are products made from petroleum, and since most lighters are disposable, over 1.5 billion each year end up in landfills or incinerators worldwide. And when choosing between a box of wood matches and a book of cardboard matches, choose the book. Wood matches come from trees, whereas most cardboard matches are made from recycled paper. If all of the cigarettes smoked every day around the world were to be lit with cardboard matches instead of wood matches, 5.5 million trees could be saved per year from going up in smoke.

Shades/Drapes

Close the curtains when it's sunny in the summer and when it's cold in the winter, and you could reduce your energy needs by up to 25 percent. If every house in America kept the curtains closed for additional insulation, the total energy saved annually would be as much as the entire nation of Japan uses in a year.

In the Utility Closet

Air Conditioner and Furnace Filters

Instead of having to replace your disposable air filter several times a year, consider buying a permanent one that can be washed and reused indefinitely. Most of these filters have lifetime warranties, so you'll save money in the long run as well as reduce the amount of waste you send to the landfill. If half of all U.S. households replaced their disposable air filters with a single reusable one, the number of air filters saved from landfills each year could blanket the entire land area of Washington, D.C.

Dry Cleaning

If you must use dry cleaners, try to go less frequently. You will not only save on drive time and fuel, you'll save plastic. Dry cleaners bunch items together into plastic garment bags, so the more items you bring at once, the better. If one in ten households took one less trip to the dry cleaners per year and saved two plastic garment bags, the plastic saved could be stitched together to make more than nine thousand hot air balloons.

Better Yet: Request no plastic garment bags, and return your paper hangers to the dry cleaners for recycling. You can also try eco-friendly dry cleaners, or wet cleaners (which use biodegradable soap).

Dryers

Clean your dryer lint screen, and don't overload the dryer. You'll save up to 5 percent on your electricity bill. If everyone did it, we'd save the energy equivalent of 350 million gallons of gasoline per year.

Better Yet: Use a clothesline when possible.

Phone Books

Recycle them.

Better Yet: Call to stop phone book delivery and then use an online telephone directory instead. Telephone books make up almost 10 percent of waste at dump sites.

Washers

Set warm wash and cold rinse cycles, and save 90 percent over the energy used when machine washing in hot water only. Together, all U.S. households could save the energy equivalent of one hundred thousand barrels of oil a day by switching from hot-hot to warm-cold cycles.

Water Heaters

Wrap your water heater in an insulating blanket to store heat. Then set the thermostat no higher than 120 degrees to conserve energy. You could save 25 percent of the energy used in your home by making these changes. If everyone did this, U.S. households would save more than $32 billion per year in energy costs.

In the Garage

Car Idling

Limit the amount of time you let your vehicle's engine run in the garage, and keep the garage door open. An idling vehicle emits twenty times more pollution than one traveling thirty-two miles per hour. There are sixty-five million garage owners in the United States. If 10 percent of garage owners were to idle their cars for just five fewer minutes per day, the total savings would be 84.5 million gallons of gas a year, enough for a million people to drive an average-size car across the country.

Car Wash

Washing your car in a commercial car wash is better for the environment than doing it yourself. Commercial car washes not only use significantly less water per wash—up to 100 gallons less—but they often recycle and reuse rinse water. If every American who currently washes a vehicle at home chose instead to go to a professional car wash—just once—up to 8.7 billion gallons of water could be saved, and some 12 billion gallons of soapy polluted water could be diverted from the country's rivers, lakes, and streams.

In the Backyard

Drip Irrigation

For flower beds and gardens, use drip irrigation or soaker hoses instead of regular sprinklers. You can save up to 70 percent of the water you would typically use because evaporation will be minimal and only the base of the plants will be receiving water as opposed to the leaves and foliage.

Existing Lawn Irrigation

Consider installing a rain sensor to override your automatic sprinkler cycle during and after rain events. Depending on the local climate, your water consumption (and your water bill) could drop up to 30 percent per year.

Hoses

Fit your garden hose with an automatic shut-off nozzle in order to prevent waste when the water is turned on and the hose is not being used. You'll save up to 6.5 gallons per minute. If just 10 percent of U.S. households attached shut-off nozzles to their hoses and the average reduction in hose usage was just thirty seconds per week, the water saved would fill over 128,000 bathtubs every day.

Lawn Care

Cut your grass so it's two inches high, and leave the clippings on the lawn. You'll spend less time mowing and raking, and you won't have to water your lawn as much. Forty percent of water in summer is allocated to outdoor usage when rates are highest. Also, less lawn care usually means using fewer chemicals that will leach into runoff water and damage local fish and bird habitats.

Pool

Cover your pool when you aren't using it and you'll cut water lost to evaporation by 90 percent and therefore the cost of replenishing it. An average-size pool with average sun and wind exposure loses approximately one thousand gallons of water per month—enough to meet the drinking water needs of a family of four for nearly a year and a half.

Outdoor Lighting

Turn off your outside lights when they're not needed. If possible, use timers or motion sensors. The average household spends about $13 per year per 100-watt bulb on electricity.

Sprinklers

Try to use your sprinklers in early morning or evening. The average lawn needs only about one hour of watering per week. In summer, outdoor water usage accounts for 40 percent of household water bills. The irrigation of U.S. lawns and landscapes claims an estimated 7.9 billion gallons of water a day—a volume that would fill fourteen billion six-packs of beer.

"We live in a world where we can get anything we want, any-place, anytime. And the faster we get it, the better. Wanna make a phone call? Speed dial. Wanna send a thank-you card? E-mail. Wanna go to the corner store? Get in the car. Our world is becoming so convenient that we take it for granted.

I've seen people drinking water out of plastic bottles and then not recycling them. That's infuriating. I know it's faster to throw it in the garbage. But if you're going to buy water individually bottled for your convenience, then all I say is, take the time and put it in the can marked 'Recycle.' It's a small thing that makes a big difference.

People don't realize how little it takes to change our world for the better. Here's something I didn't know: I thought that all the oil in our oceans was caused by tanker spills. It's not. I learned that twenty-four million out of the twenty-nine million gallons of oil that go into North America's oceans each year are caused by human activities. Twenty-four million gallons of oil! That's crazy! I usually use it by the tablespoon. What happens is we pour cooking oil into our sinks, top off our gas tanks, and hose down grease from our cars into storm drains, then it goes into our oceans.

We can fix that. Put your cooking oil into a container and throw it in the garbage. Don't top off your gas tank. Use drip pans when you work on your car, and take used oil and anti-freeze to recycling centers. These are things we can do. And I'm also going to talk to Richard Simmons about his oil usage. Maybe we can bring those numbers down.

entertainment

Sex, Drugs, Rock 'n' Roll, and Recycling

THE BIG PICTURE

Having fun means tons of trash. Literally. Empties and cigarette butts are good reminders of what's bad. More than eighty billion cans and bottles that could be recycled are just lying around as trash. Trillions of cigarette butts litter the planet. And even if you don't party like a rock star, waste from having a good time can add up. Take a parade. The famous Tournament of Roses Parade attracts half a million spectators, as well as 100 tons of trash. And that doesn't even include tailgating!

Speaking of watching trash pile up—every year, 2 million books, 350 million magazines, and 24 billion newspapers are thrown away. And you thought no one read anymore! Sure, newspapers may be going the way of eight-track cassettes, but new technology isn't helping old habits: One hundred thousand CDs are thrown away each month, along with 5.5 million boxes of software. That's enough to make even Bill Gates shed a tear.

But the real problem faced by the entertainment industry is energy. Not only do live events sap energy for lights, sound, amps, and video screens, but just about everything related to watching and listening takes wattage. One live event can burn through as much electricity in a few hours as seven hundred households use all year. Even that, though, pales in comparison with what's at the top of the "e-waste" mountain: batteries. The average person owns about two button batteries and ten normal (A, AA, AAA, C, D, 9V, and so on) batteries and throws out about eight household batteries per year. Some three billion batteries are sold annually in the United States, averaging about thirty-two per family or ten per person.

Do the math and you'll see that almost as many batteries are thrown away each year as are purchased. The problem isn't just about waste, the problem is the mercury, lead, and other toxic chemicals that batteries contain. Considering that most hazardous waste is incinerated, well, you don't have to be a chemist to figure out that a lot of pollution is being created.

Water, too, runs dry when it comes to entertainment. It takes 1,500 gallons of water to make just a single drive-through order: hamburger, French fries, and a soda. This includes the water needed to grow potatoes, the grain for the bun and the cattle, and everything for the soda.

Gulp.

Keeping all that in mind, we've created the "Simple Steps" to be just that. Taking into account all the points of the Big Picture, they give you the biggest impact with the least amount of effort.

The Simple Steps

1. Use fewer paper napkins—everywhere. There's no need to grab a huge stack of napkins from the concession stand when you know you'll use only one or two. Each American consumes an average of 2,200 standard two-ply napkins per year, or the equivalent of just over six of these napkins per day. If everyone in the United States used an average of one fewer napkin per day, more than a billion pounds of napkins could be saved from landfills each year. A stack of napkins this size could fill the entire Empire State Building.

2. Buy rechargeable batteries, and you'll save money over the long term. A single rechargeable battery can replace up to one thousand single-use alkaline batteries over its lifetime. Americans throw out approximately 179,000 tons of batteries per year.

3. Drink tap water when dining out. You can save as much as $7 for a bottle of water, and it may be safer to drink. Tap water is more strictly regulated than bottled water. If everyone drank tap instead of bottled water in the United States, it would save about $8 billion—about as much as the United States spends each year in drought response. It also would help prevent plastic waste: Sixty million water bottles are tossed each day in the United States.

THE LITTLE THINGS

Albums

About one million vinyl LPs are still sold each year in the United States. So instead of just tossing your old records in the trash, you may be able to sell them for about $10 each. While the LPs can be put into the recycle bin, recycling takes a lot more energy than you'll spend dropping off your old LPs at a nearby used-record store.

Books

Use the library, or buy secondhand books. Consider sharing the ones you have with friends or donating them rather than throwing them away. About three billion new books are sold per year, requiring four hundred thousand trees to be chopped down.

Candy

Buy loose, unwrapped candy from the bin, if you can. Many candy wrappers contain chemicals that make them stain- and water-resistant but also make them difficult to recycle.

Compact Discs

Download tunes instead of purchasing them at the store. The average price of a CD is about $15, whereas an album download is only about $10. Each month, more than forty-five tons of CDs become obsolete— outdated or unwanted—and end up in landfills.

DVDs

Rent DVDs instead of buying them. Depending upon how much you watch one, you could save money. The average movie rents for about $4, while the average new DVD sells for more than $16. You also won't have to worry about contributing to their trash pile: One hundred thousand DVDs and CDs are thrown away each month. If you do own DVDs and want to discard them, donate them to a local library or thrift store, or look for a DVD recycling center.

Gift Wrap

Skip gift wrapping altogether, reuse ribbons, or use other paper materials like old newspapers or old maps. If each family reused just two feet of holiday ribbon each year, thirty-eight thousand miles' worth would be saved. That's enough to tie a bow around the entire planet.

Invitations

Use electronic invitations, or choose "chlorine-free postconsumer recycled paper" for your party invitations. Online invitations eliminate stationery and mailing costs, and postconsumer recycled paper costs about the same as primary fiber paper. Better use of paper could allow the world's wood consumption to be reduced by 50 percent and possibly by as much as 80 percent or more.

Magazines

If you subscribe to your favorite magazines instead of buying them from a newsstand, you'll get the convenience of delivery and will save 75 percent or more off the newsstand price. Sixty percent of most magazines at the newsstand aren't sold and have to be hauled off to the trash dump—a waste of time, money, and energy.

MP3 Players

Recycle or return to the manufacturer your old MP3 players. Some companies give customers up to 10 percent off their next purchase when they return their old players. About 40 percent of all the lead in U.S. landfills comes from improperly discarded electronic waste, which can result in toxic pollution of the air and groundwater. So be sure to seek out an e-waste collector or recycling service.

Newspapers

Subscribe to and recycle your newspapers. Newspaper subscribers can save about 50 percent off the cover price, as well as a trip to the newsstand. Each year, ten million tons of newspapers are still tossed into landfills and aren't recycled. If just half of these were recycled, it would save seventy-five million trees.

Placeware

Use porcelain plates, silverware, and glasses instead of plastic and paper.

Each year, forty billion plastic utensils are thrown into landfills across the country. Besides waste, you can save money, too. Using your own utensils, glasses, and flatware is free, whereas the cost of plastic plates, forks, knives, and cups for a total of fifty meals could add up to $100.

Popcorn

Share your popcorn when you're at the movies instead of buying multiple cartons or bags. You'll save money and packaging. Americans today consume seventeen billion quarts of popcorn each year (fifty-four quarts per person), 30 percent of which are eaten at movie theaters, sporting events, entertainment arenas, amusement parks, and other recreational centers. If half the people shared their popcorn at these events, we could save the paper packaging for more than 2.5 billion quart-size servings.

Restaurants

Take home what you don't eat, and ask for as little packaging as possible. Use it for Fido or as compost for your lawn or garden. This reduces food scraps and the disposal costs that restaurants bear. Twelve percent of landfills are food scraps, and one-quarter of all food produced in the United States is wasted.

Soda

If you have the choice, buy soda from the fountain in a paper cup instead of from a can or plastic bottle. You'll reduce the amount of aluminum cans and plastic bottles that are wasted. More paper (48 percent) is recycled and recovered to make new products than aluminum soda cans (43.9 percent) or plastic soda bottles (25 percent).

Televisions

Unplug your TV when it's not in use. You'll save money and energy. Between 10 and 15 percent of a TV's energy is still used when it's powered "off." TV use accounts for more than 10 percent of household electricity bills. The average household in America owns more than two TVs. If every home just unplugged their TV sets when they weren't being used, we'd save more than $1 billion per year in energy bills. To make this easier, try connecting your TV to an outlet that is connected to a wall switch.

Tickets

Buy your movie and event tickets online or via telephone and print them at home. You'll save time and paper waste. Print-at-home tickets use plain copy paper, which is easier to make into recycled paper than the paperboard used for printed tickets. Some 1.4 billion movie tickets alone are sold in the United States annually—and almost every one of them goes to waste.

Videocameras

Sell, donate, or recycle your videocamera rather than tossing it. Consumers will throw out about four hundred million electronics this year. E-waste is the fastest-growing segment of municipal waste.

" It used to be that people who cared about the environment were called granola heads and tree huggers and treated like kooks. Now they're called visionaries, and tree hugger is a great eco-website, and maybe granola head is, too.

At an early age, I felt the power of nature growing up in a Los Angeles of orange groves; plenty of green space; clean, clear air; fully alive. I worked summers in Yosemite National Park, and its beauty stopped me in my tracks. Maybe it was the experience of watching Los Angeles paved over and streets coughing brown air, but I wanted to protect this feeling I got from being in nature and the solace and inspiration I found in it.

But truthfully, I stumbled upon my activism the way lots of people do. The government had plans to build a six-lane highway in my backyard, through a pristine Utah canyon, and ruin it forever, disrupt ecosystems, pollute it all, including the air my kids would breathe and the water they'd drink. So I locked arms with local activists to fight it; we held them off for the time being, and therein started a now forty-year quest to try to make a difference for the environment and for the future.

It doesn't matter if you're a Democrat, Republican, or Independent, as the environment and things like global warming know no political affiliation, but it's true that they often become the political football and are treated as political sport. Politics will always be part of the equation. Whom we elect to office on every level will always play into it all. The whole political system can be irritatingly sluggish, stalemated, and the barriers can seem insurmountable. But then little pockets of inspiration slowly begin opening up, joining together, and building a collective force that can suddenly give way to tremendous change.

What has always given me hope is that small steps can lead to sea change. As important as is the big picture, there's profound power in pulling it down to a manageable scale, to bringing it home, right down into our communities, and taking action with available solutions. The little things count as much as the big things when enough people are doing them. And there's something very positive, very democratic, about the people gathering together in our common interest. How we treat the earth says much about us as a society, about our spirit and strength as a nation. I am extremely optimistic that we, the people, will turn the tide.

That's why this book is so important. And that's where you come in.

It's your future. 〞

travel

The Family Vacation That Ate the Planet

THE BIG PICTURE

Tourism is the third largest retail business in the United States, behind automotive dealers and food stores. It's a $1.3 trillion industry. That means people spend an average of $3.4 billion a day on travel-related goods and services. Daily, some 2.6 million hotels rooms are rented and about 30,000 commercial flights are taken. Almost everyone in America—91 percent of adults—takes a vacation to spend thirteen days a year getting away from their day-to-day routines. Fifteen percent of American travelers fly (96 percent stay in the United States, 4 percent go overseas), 82 percent drive, and 3 percent travel by bus, train, or boat.

All of this moving about translates into a lot of energy consumption. It's the biggest trade-off for all that fun. And it's a big trade-off for work, too, as business travel makes up a huge portion of air travel.

In fact, air travel is fast becoming the largest contributor of greenhouse gas emissions. More people are flying than ever before; about three-quarters of a billion people fly around the United States each year. This puts more toxins in the air at higher altitudes, which can be more damaging to the air and ozone layer than ground-level emissions.

Beyond travel, people somehow waste bucketloads of water while they're on vacation: The tourism industry uses 93.9 billion gallons of water per year, 4 percent of the total U.S. commercial consumption. The average hotel room consumes 209 gallons of water per day. That's almost as much as an entire U.S. household uses daily!

But it's not just the consumption of water while people are on vacation that can pose a problem. Sometimes it's the oceans, lakes, rivers, and wetlands that are used for recreation. When boating, swimming, kayaking, tubing, or snorkeling, tourists can damage ecosystems by littering, polluting, or stepping on fragile aquatic habitats (such as coral reefs). The same thing can happen while hiking. One or two tourists may not cause visible harm, but hundreds over time can do substantial damage to natural areas as well as to feeding patterns and wildlife. This is important considering that camping is the number one outdoor vacation activity in America.

Keeping all that in mind, we've created the "Simple Steps" to be just that. Taking into account all the points of the Big Picture, they give you the biggest impact with the least amount of effort.

The Simple Steps

1. Use the same linens and towels in your hotel room throughout your stay. You probably don't change your sheets and towels every day at home, so why do it while you're away? The average hotel room consumes more than two hundred gallons of water per day, or as much as your entire household typically uses in a day. Trimming the amount of water used by washing sheets and towels can save up to 40 percent of a hotel's water use.

2. Travel in groups. Put four people in a taxi instead of two, and double the fuel efficiency.

Better Yet: Take a bus. For the amount of fuel it takes for you to go a mile in a car, you can go five miles in a bus.

3. **Pack lightly.** Every additional ten pounds per traveler requires an additional 350 million gallons of jet fuel per year, which is enough to keep a 747 flying continuously for ten years.

THE LITTLE THINGS

Travel Planning

Adventure Travel

Ninety-eight million people within the last five years hiked, biked, white-water rafted, and kayaked all over the planet. Adventure travel forces travelers to become actively engaged with new cultures and environments, as well as hopefully becoming more aware and respectful of the outdoors.

Camera

Use a digital camera instead of one that needs film. Some 686 million rolls of film are processed each year, and the solutions used to make the prints often contain hazardous chemicals that require special treatment and disposal. Avoid using disposable cameras. Despite the claim on the box that they're recycled, more than half end up in the trash.

Cruise

Try an eco-friendly sailing cruise rather than a vacation aboard a cruise ship. Sailing cruises carry fewer passengers and don't disrupt ports and seas nearly as much as giant cruise ships, which can spill oil and sewage and disturb fish habitats. Nearly twelve million people take cruises each year, most from North America, using some 170 cruise liners. A single ship consumes several thousand gallons of fuel—per hour.

Eco-Tourism

Try eco-tourism, which focuses on local culture and promotes environmental awareness. You'll get a different perspective and potentially save money. Eco-travel features destinations that aren't overcrowded or overrun. It draws attention to environmentally sensitive areas and pumps approximately $250 billion into the economies of developing countries.

Guidebooks

Research your trip online, and print out only the pages you'll actually need to reference. You'll save time, money, and paper waste. With close to one million guidebooks printed annually, but just 18 percent being recycled, more than eight hundred thousand travel books go to waste every year.

Hotels

Look into visiting eco-friendly hotels. They offer prices that rival regular hotels but have facilities and programs that conserve water and energy. You might just sleep easier knowing that you're helping to use 20 percent less water and 40 percent less energy than you'd be using if you were staying in a standard hotel room.

Luggage Tags

Use the tag that came with your luggage set. You'll save time at the airline check-in counter as well as paper. If every traveler in the United States stopped using paper luggage tags for each of their trips, sixty million sheets of paper could be saved per year.

Maps

Use online maps instead of paper maps, or use your car's satellite navigation. Online maps are free, and if you have to print them out, you'll be able to better recycle the paper when you're done with them. Map paper is particularly difficult—sometimes impossible—to recycle because of all the ink used. If you've got old maps, reuse them as gift wrapping instead of just throwing them out.

Ticketing

Use e-tickets instead of paper tickets. You can save as much as $30 per ticket, and the airline industry could save as much as $3 billion annually by eliminating paper tickets altogether. With the paper saved, you'd have enough to provide boarding passes for all of the people in India.

Time of Year

Try traveling during the off-season. Traveling out of season can reduce travel costs by 40 percent, and you'll avoid crowds and lines at sites and attractions. If you travel to major cities and destination spots, you'll create less of an impact on the planet by reducing traffic in urban areas—by as much as 22 percent—and thus reduce vehicle carbon emissions by 14 percent. When there are fewer people in one spot, it reduces congestion.

Toiletries

Pack your own shampoo, soap, and toothpaste instead of relying on those provided by most hotels. You'll get the product you want rather than some odd scented gel, and you'll create less plastic waste. A single three-hundred-room hotel in Las Vegas uses more than 150,000 plastic bottles of shampoo per year.

Leaving Home

Appliances

Unplug your appliances, where possible, when you leave home. Residential consumers in the United States spend more than $5 billion annually on standby power alone—about 5 percent of all electricity consumed in the country.

Lights

Use timers on your lights instead of leaving on the porch light. The average household spends about $13 per year per hundred-watt bulb on electricity. If every home in America used a timer for twelve hours a day instead of letting their lights burn 24/7 while on vacation, we could save $187 million in energy costs!

Mail

Stop delivery of your mail while you're away. You'll save the post office from having to transport your mail and avoid having friends travel to store it for you. Because the U.S. Postal Service delivers approximately 212 billion letters, advertisements, periodicals, and packages a year, every penny of transportation costs adds up—so much so that just a one-cent increase in fuel prices costs the post office $8 million.

Newspapers

Stop delivery of your newspaper while you're away. You'll stop waste and save money. Many newspapers will credit your account for the days you're away. Paper is the biggest source of waste to landfills, and about 30 percent of all newspapers are thrown in the trash, not recycled.

Shades

Close them when you leave the house. Depending on the season, keeping your curtains closed will insulate heat or keep your home cool.

These steps could help you reduce your energy needs by up to 25 percent. If every home in America closed the curtains when it was sunny in the summer or cold in the winter, we'd save as much energy as Japan uses over the same amount of time.

Thermostat

When you're away, adjust your thermostat to fifty degrees during cold months and to eighty-five degrees in hot months. Depending upon how long you're gone, you could save up to $100 per year in energy costs related to heating and cooling your home when you aren't there. The United States uses $1 million worth of energy every minute. You can help to lower that by turning the dial.

Getting There

Baggage

If possible, take just a carry-on and you'll save time at the airport. The average airline passenger waits between twenty and thirty minutes at the carousel to pick up luggage. Carousels operate off of electric motors that sap energy. Electric motors account for 70 percent of industrial energy use; carry-ons can help reduce their drain.

Check-In

Try self-service, and use print-at-home tickets. Self-check-in saves the airlines $1 billion per year, and you save time in the ticket line. Fifty-nine percent of people check in through the airline's main counter, which takes an average of nineteen minutes; 18 percent use a self-check-in kiosk, which averages eight minutes; 10 percent check in at curbside, which averages thirteen minutes; and 5 percent of passengers obtain their boarding pass through the Internet, which lets them go straight to the security checkpoint. Moreover, printing your tickets at home means you can print on recycled paper. Cardboard boarding passes handed out at the gate are almost always more difficult to recycle because of the ink used and, in some cases, the magnetic strips placed on the back.

Hybrid Car Service

Try a hybrid taxi. If the entire New York City taxi fleet were converted to hybrids, the result in terms of reduced exhaust emissions would be the equivalent of taking twenty-four thousand cars off the road.

Transportation

Share rides to the airport and split your fare with a fellow passenger. You'll also help reduce pollution and traffic congestion. Airlines carry about 750 million passengers per year in the United States, which means that 750 million people need to be transported to the airport on each end of their trip. If just an additional 10 percent of travelers could share a $30 ride with one other person, the total annual savings would top $1 billion.

At the Hotel

Lights

Turn them off when you leave the room. Seventy-five percent of the energy in a hotel room is used when the bathroom lights are left on for more than two hours—mostly when it's unoccupied!

Plugs/Adapters

Unplug your adapters when you're on the road. Plugs and adapters often do not match wattage requirements exactly and can "leak" energy. In the United States, failing to unplug adapters can waste 5 percent of the energy used. Overseas, there is even more waste—between 10 and 15 percent in Europe and Japan.

Washing Clothes

Wait until you get home to wash your clothes. It's far less expensive. You'll pay several dollars for each article of clothing the hotel launders for you. The hotel industry uses 16,863 gallons of water per room per year. In fact, an average 150-room hotel uses as many resources in a week as one hundred families use in a year.

Sightseeing/Getting Around

Car Rentals

Try a hybrid car or a more fuel-efficient vehicle. A hybrid rental can go three times as far as a standard sedan on a single tank of gas. There are 1.7 million rental cars in the United States. If every one of them were a hybrid, more than nine million gallons of gasoline would be saved—per fill-up!

Locations

Seek out locations that aren't overexposed, overcrowded, or in environmentally sensitive areas. Overcrowding in already densely populated areas can lead to increased pollution by wastewater, garbage, heating, noise, and traffic emissions. Rome's Colosseum was partially destroyed because of increased air pollution due to traffic and tourism.

Paths

Stay on paths when you tour or hike. In delicate habitats, vegetation destruction and rock slides can easily be caused by the trampling of too many people.

Souvenirs

Buy souvenirs from local manufacturers rather than trinkets made somewhere else. It helps support the economies of the sites you're visiting.

Water Bottles

Use and refill a single water bottle, thermos, or canteen when you travel. The average person in the United States drinks eight ounces of bottled water per day. Considering that plastic is derived from petroleum, it takes 1.5 million barrels of oil annually to satisfy America's demand for bottled water. If this oil were converted to gasoline, the total could fuel five hundred thousand station wagons to take their families on coast-to-coast road trips.

"There are two activities in my personal life that give me limitless amounts of joy. They are, quite simply, driving my electric car and making a trip to the hazardous waste facility.

First off, driving an electric car could not be more fun. People are constantly coming up to me and asking a range of questions. How does it drive? Great, surprisingly peppy. How does it work? You charge it at home with a charging unit that's installed and charges overnight. What kind of range do you have? I can go up to eighty miles on one charge, which for city driving means I can go an entire week before I charge it again. If I lose weight, I can go even farther! In fact, I constantly tell people that if you could drive this car, you wouldn't want to drive another car. There's no emissions, it's quiet, and for the cost of the electricity (which comes out to roughly thirty cents a gallon), there's no wonder the auto industry stopped making and started destroying these cars. But they can't hold back the tide. They're going to be coming back, and if you get a chance, purchase one; it makes your heart smile when you drive.

Now when I pull up to the hazardous waste facility with my EV . . . look out. There's nothing more exciting than emptying my garage of used paints, old batteries, any old appliance or piece of electronics, and loading up my electric car. It's a great feeling that we, as a family, are not putting any of those items in a landfill. That they are being disposed of properly. And here's the best part! You pull up to the collection station and never have to get out of your car!! The people working on-site ask you to unlock your trunk and they do all the rest.

It's funny how these small things, these actions, add up to be big things."

communication/technology

I Can't Hang Out with You Because I Have to Call, Text, IM, and E-Mail My Friends All Day

THE BIG PICTURE

Listen up. The communication revolution is crowding the world with devices. You can get a cell phone signal in the middle of Africa or e-mail your friends on your laptop computer while flying over the Atlantic Ocean. Technology is great, but along with it comes a price: e-waste.

Electronic waste is the fastest-growing segment of municipal land-fills around the world. And it's not "good" waste, either. Computer monitors contain lead. Batteries hold lithium. And then there's the zinc, mercury, and copper that go into the electronic guts of today's machinery. When burned, this stuff poisons the air we breathe. When left in piles, the toxins seep into the ground and contaminate the soil and groundwater.

The problem is massive.

About 130 million cell phones get tossed every year. Soon, there will be as many discarded every year as are purchased. Considering there are about 2 billion cell phones on the planet, that's a lot of little screens.

Now add 50 million computer monitors and you have a pile that, if stacked one on top of another, climbs past the most distant satellite orbiting the earth.

And this doesn't even take into account all the dusty, worn-out fax machines, computers, and cell phones sitting in people's basements and attics. According to some estimates, there are another 2 billion of these types of electronic products that have yet to make it to the trash.

Not that you can just throw out those electronic products with the trash. Many states have laws that require people to dispose of computers, televisions, cell phones, and other electronic devices as they would hazardous waste, through special collection agencies. In Europe, certain types of electronics are banned from even being sold.

Unfortunately, the final resting place for many trashed products is the third world—places like India and Africa. But this only shifts the burden. In these places, the hazards of electronic waste disposal are exacerbated, because toxic items are often incinerated, sending fumes into the air . . . fumes that can travel and land right back here in this country.

Nasty.

There are leaks like that, things you can't see, all over the place in the electronics world: Your power strips are sucking energy all the while they're on. Even your e-mail uses power you cannot see.

What is in plain sight, however, is just how much communication and technology have invaded our lives. The average U.S. household has twenty-four different electronic devices—computers, cell phones, televisions, VCRs, DVD players, answering machines, and printers, among other things.

Keeping all that in mind, we've created the "Simple Steps" to be just that. Taking into account all the points of the Big Picture, they give you the biggest impact with the least amount of effort.

The Simple Steps

1. **Recycle your cellular phone.** Donate your phone to a charity or sell it to a third-party recycler. You can often take a tax deduction for the phone's value or get hard money for it from a recycler. Less than 1 percent of cell phones are currently recycled, and there are five hundred million used cell phones not being used in the United States alone!

2. **Unplug your power.** Ten percent of the electricity used in your home is burned by communication devices and appliances—when they are turned off! If every U.S. household just unplugged its computers and cell phone chargers when they were not being used, collectively we'd save over $100 million—enough to provide free health care to every low-income child under the age of five in the state of California.

3. **Download your software.** Most software comes on a compact disc, and more than thirty billion compact discs of all types are sold annually—enough to wrap around the earth. Put another way, that's five CDs produced each year for each person on the planet. With more than one billion unwanted computer disks being thrown away per year, that's a huge mountain of waste, not to mention the packaging material—fifty-five million boxes. Most software can be downloaded online.

THE LITTLE THINGS

Answering Machines

Use voice mail instead. Answering machines guzzle energy 24/7. When they stop functioning, they become hazardous waste in the nation's landfills. If all answering machines in U.S. homes were eventually replaced by voice mail services, the annual energy savings would total nearly two billion kilowatt-hours. The reduction in air pollution related to this decrease in energy use would be equivalent to removing 250,000 cars from the road for a year.

Auto Switching

Try "auto switching" power strips. They shut down when the primary appliance is turned off and can save up to four kilowatt-hours per day of energy. If every home in America switched to more efficient power strips, we could save enough energy to power forty thousand homes for a year.

Computers

Use the power management mode. You can save up to $75 per year merely by enabling the low-power sleep modes on your monitors and CPUs.

Digital

Go digital on all your products. Cell phones and even televisions are going to be mandated to use digital signals as of 2009, making all television sets that rely only on an antenna without a digital tuner unable to receive television broadcasts without an external digital broadcast receiver. So if you buy a broadcast-only (analog) TV, you're just going to have to toss it eventually. There are still twenty million households that use broadcast-only TVs, which will sooner than later end up in landfills.

Discs

Use Blu-ray Discs if you can. The format offers more than five times the storage capacity of traditional compact discs. Blu-ray Discs are half made of paper, so they can even be shredded, making them easier to dispose of and recycle than traditional CDs.

Headsets

Try *not* to use a wireless headset for your phone. They use batteries. More than 350 million tons of button-size batteries—the type used for headsets—are sold every year. These contain mercury, lead, and zinc, which can pollute the air and water if disposed of improperly. Never throw out batteries with the trash. Always take them to a local hazardous waste disposal site.

High-Speed Internet
Try to use faster Internet access. It saves time and ultimately money and energy. High-speed access users, on average, accomplish more than double the number of tasks online compared with dial-up users. That means it would take more than an hour to do via dial-up what you could do in thirty minutes via broadband. Based on a full day's use, you could save more than $30 per year in energy costs by increasing your Internet efficiency and turning off your computer when it's not in use.

Messaging
If you can, send a text message or e-mail from a handheld device or cell phone, instead of from a computer, especially quick, one-line notes. You'll save yourself time and conserve energy. Compared to sending a text message, e-mailing and text messaging from a computer uses more than thirty times the electricity per message.

Pagers
Don't just toss them in the trash. Try reusing the batteries for low-use items, like remote controls or clocks. More than forty-five million people had pagers in 1998, before most switched to cell phones. That means ninety million batteries (pagers use two) could possibly be saved and used for channel surfing instead.

Personal Digital Assistants
Choose ones that are RoHS (Restriction of Hazardous Substances Directive) compliant—or have reduced amounts of hazardous materials. About ten million personal digital assistants (PDAs) are sold annually in

the United States (not including smart phones). The same issues as cell phones apply to PDAs: The lead they contain can seep out of landfills and contaminate groundwater. If the tubes are crushed and burned, they emit toxic fumes into the air. Proper disposal of your PDA and other electronic devices can help reduce the concentration of toxic waste sent to landfills. Currently, 40 percent of the lead and 70 percent of the heavy metals in landfills are attributed to e-waste.

Power Strips

Turn off your power strips when they're not in use. The average American household continuously leaks about fifty watts of electricity. Eliminating that trickle would save $1 billion a year in wasted electricity.

Power Usage

Use smaller items that draw less power, such as laptops. Many laptops now are even less expensive than many desktops, and they use far less energy: more than 50 percent less. If every computer user in the United States used a laptop, we'd save about $2.5 billion in energy costs.

" Some things are important for the world to know...like how long I shower. Seriously. I take a three-minute shower. It's three minutes, or as short as possible, for a good reason, however. I even brush wash—brush my teeth while I shower. Now here's why: I found out that every two minutes in the shower uses as much water as a person in Africa uses for everything in their life for a whole day—drinking, bathing, cooking, and cleaning...everything! When you become aware of all the things you do, and the effect those things have, you want to make small changes. Like with water. So now you know why I brush and wash at the same time. When I found out that my cell phone charger still uses energy when it's plugged in and it's not being used, I began unplugging it. When I found out that I could use less gas and get better mileage with a hybrid car, I bought a Prius.

It all goes back to awareness and knowing better and then making a simple shift in habit. When you're a kid, your mom tells you to clean your room and turn off the lights. So you listen to her and you do it. (Well, sometimes.) That becomes a shift in habit, something you do unconsciously. Obviously, when I learn about something new that I can do in my everyday life that makes a whole lot of sense and can help the environment, I do it. Eventually, it just becomes second nature. If we all begin to learn from one another and share some of the things we do, we just might be able to affect the world for the better through these little rituals. In a curious way, this would be a great wave of awareness: doing the right thing without being told to or having to think why.

Now, about my baths... "

school

A Mind Is a Terrible Thing to Waste,
but Waste Is a Terrific Thing to Mind

THE BIG PICTURE

There are 75.5 million students who attend school in the United States, and their waste is something to be examined in and of itself.

U.S. colleges and universities create about 3.6 million tons of waste a year, which amounts to 2 percent of the country's total waste stream. Add to that the waste from high schools, elementary schools, and even kindergartens, and you have a problematic equation.

Almost half of all school waste comes from paper: writing paper, drawing paper, copy paper, tests, exams—paper and more paper. A lot of it is recycled, but a lot of it isn't. More than half of it, in fact, is just thrown out with the garbage.

Meanwhile, millions of servings of food go to waste. Just one elementary school creates 18,760 pounds of lunch waste per year. But it would be better if kids ate less, too. The childhood obesity rate has more than doubled since 1970 for preschool children between two and five years old and adolescents between twelve and nineteen years old. It has more than tripled for children between six and eleven years old.

About nine million children over the age of six are considered obese. Teenagers are no better. Twenty-three percent say they eat a great deal of junk food in a typical week; 61 percent say they eat some; 14 percent eat hardly any; and only 2 percent eat none. Here's where that affects the environment: 67 percent of kids say they buy junk food or soda from vending machines at school. That means more packaging and more waste.

Obviously, students need to be taught different habits. But some things are beyond their control, like how their classrooms are heated, cooled, or lighted. Schools use more than $6 billion annually in energy, with 25 percent, or about $1.5 billion, wasted because of energy inefficiency. This equates to enough money to hire thirty thousand new teachers.

Practicing conservation isn't brain surgery . . . it's turning off the lights.

Keeping all that in mind, we've created the "Simple Steps" to be just that. Taking into account all the points of the Big Picture, they give you the biggest impact with the least amount of effort.

The Simple Steps

1. **Pack a waste-free lunch**. Eliminate plastic bags, plastic utensils, disposable containers, paper napkins, and those brown paper bags. Instead use a reusable lunchbox, reusable drink containers, cloth napkins, and silverware. You could save $250 a year and as much weight in waste as the average nine-year-old!

2. **Walk to school.** Only 31 percent of children who live less than one mile from school walk there. Half of all students go to school by car. If just 6 percent of those students who go by car walked, it would save 1.5 million dropoffs and pickups—and sixty thousand gallons of gasoline—a day!

3. **Use both sides of your plain paper, and recycle.** Paper is the biggest form of waste that comes from schools. Every ton, or 220,000 sheets, of paper that is recycled saves approximately seventeen trees. The average school tosses thirty-eight tons of paper per year, or more than 8 million sheets!

THE LITTLE THINGS

Getting There

Bicycle
Only 2.5 percent of students who live within two miles of school get there via bicycle. Still, by not taking a bus or a car, those six hundred thousand students are saving almost one hundred thousand gallons of gasoline—a day.

Bus
If you can, hop a bus rather than take a car to school. School buses account for an estimated ten billion student trips each year, while reporting fewer traffic accidents than private transportation. You can travel more than five miles on a full bus with the energy it takes to go just one mile in a car.

Carpooling
Carpool, and save time and money. On a typical day, the average mother with school-age children spends sixty-six minutes driving—taking more than five trips to and from home and covering twenty-nine miles. If more moms carpooled, it would save them all that time and gas driving. It also would reduce congestion, which costs Americans $78 billion a year in wasted fuel and lost time.

In the Classroom

Blackboard Erasers
Don't clap erasers to clean them, and be sure to clean them outdoors. Electronic equipment in classrooms with blackboards has to be cleaned twice as often, and rooms with chalk dust cost more to clean.

Blackboards
Request that whiteboards be used instead of blackboards. Chalk creates dust on the hands and on the surrounding media, sparking allergies and causing computer damage. Using nontoxic dry-erase markers on whiteboards eliminates chalk dust damage.

Chalk
Request dust-free chalk. It limits potential exposure to airborne particles that aggravate asthma and other respiratory illnesses. Asthma affects over five million school-age children and youth in the United States— about one out of every eleven students—and it's a leading cause of school absenteeism.

Crayons
Avoid crayons made from paraffin wax, which is derived from petroleum. Instead, try using crayons made from soybean oil, which have the added benefit of being nontoxic. America is the largest producer of soybeans in the world. From this we could produce well over one trillion crayons—without tapping oil supplies!

Markers
Markers can contain harsh chemicals (evidenced by their strong smell). Because toxic chemicals can leak into the groundwater from the landfills at which they're disposed, it's better to use markers that are water based and have nontoxic ink with refillable heads.

Pencils

Use pencils made from recycled material and those packed in light-weight or recyclable packaging. Pencils can be made from all sorts of things that would otherwise end up in our waste stream—like furniture, old money, and paper. Pencils account for about $121 million worth of purchases every year, and all could potentially be made from recycled materials.

Pens

Use refillable pens. Pen refills cost as little as $1 each, priced almost the same as disposable ones. Pens are often tossed into the garbage and not recycled or reused. Their components and packaging are made from nonrenewable resources and can contain environmentally damaging chemicals. Every year, Americans discard 1.6 billion pens. Placed end to end, they would stretch more than 150,000 miles—equivalent to crossing the Pacific Ocean from Los Angeles to Tokyo more than twenty-five times!

Schoolbooks

Buy used textbooks and sell them back when you're done. You'll make money and save money (as much as 85 percent). About $10 billion worth of schoolbooks—kindergarten through college—are sold every year. Recycling just 1 percent of these books would save enough money to send more than four thousand students to a four-year public college for free!

Temperature

Ask teachers to keep classroom temperatures between sixty-nine and seventy-three degrees. It will save energy and improve the learning environment. In classrooms kept at controlled temperatures, students scored higher on tests and exams than they did at much colder or warmer temperatures. Every degree of temperature saved also means a cost savings per schoolroom of 2 percent on utility bills.

At Lunch

Food Donation
Seek out a food donation program for your school instead of discarding unused cafeteria food. If every chartered school (there are 3,600 of them) participated in a donation program for an entire school year, the savings could feed one meal to more than two million starving people.

Food Types
Sandwiches, fresh fruit, fresh vegetables, and treats packed in reusable lunch containers are healthy alternatives to cafeteria and prepackaged foods. Also, they can be bought in larger quantities, saving money and packaging. The packaging can be left at home for reuse or recycling.

Gum
Dispose of your gum in the trash, not on the ground (or under your desk). The average American chews up to 190 sticks of gum each year. In all, those 57 billion sticks could add up to a gum patch four miles wide and six miles long.

Recycling
Practice recycling, and encourage your teachers and fellow students to recycle as well. By recycling 90 percent of the waste that would other-wise go to a landfill, a single elementary school could save $6,000 per year in landfill disposal costs.

Vending Machines
Try not to buy drinks and snacks from vending machines. Forty-three percent of elementary schools, 89.4 percent of middle/junior high schools, and 98.2 percent of senior high schools have vending machines, school stores, canteens, or snack bars. Items sold from these sources are usually preserved with plastic packaging, a big source of landfill waste.

Homework

Library Books

Try using a digital library or the World Wide Web instead of traveling to your local branch to do research. You'll save time and money. The circulation of books from public libraries is 1.9 billion a year, or about 7 items checked out per person. If every American checked out and researched online a single book a year, we would save three hundred million trips to the bookshelves.

School Supplies

Adhesive Notes

Look for paper notes made of 100 percent recycled fiber and at least 30 percent postconsumer content. Sales of adhesive notes are estimated at about $1 billion per year. A pack of one hundred sells for about $1.25, which means some eighty billion little stick 'em notes are stuck somewhere every year.

Binders

Try using binders made from recycled materials (like paper, boards, steel, and so on) and reusing them year after year. If 80 percent of students did so, the materials saved could build a binder with an area of 1,240 acres—larger than the entire campus of the University of California at Berkeley.

File Folders

Try to use 100 percent recycled file folders with postconsumer recycled fiber. This fiber is derived from paper that is recovered from the waste stream. By buying recycled instead of virgin paper in general, you'll reduce solid waste from the materials by almost 50 percent. You can also flip folders inside out and reuse them. And that's important when paper makes up about half the trash.

Notebooks

Try using wire-bound notebooks with 20 percent postconsumer fiber. They're cheap and help reduce landfill waste. A paper mill uses 20 percent less energy to make paper from recycled material than it does to make paper from fresh lumber. For every one hundred pounds of trash we throw away, thirty-nine pounds is paper.

Paper

Try to buy recycled paper and avoid paper that contains chlorine. Postconsumer recycled paper (which is paper that is used and then tossed, as opposed to preconsumer recycled paper, which is made out of scraps and trimmings) requires 44 percent less energy to produce, reducing greenhouse gas emissions by 37 percent and producing 48 percent less solid waste. If we reduced paper use of all kinds by half, we'd clear space currently occupied by more than one thousand landfills.

Paper Clips

Recycle your paper clips, or just reuse the one you have! Enough paper clips are produced each year to hand every person in the world at least three. For every one hundred thousand paper clips produced, only twenty thousand are used to hold together paper. The rest aren't being used!

Plastic

Avoid products that contain polyvinyl chloride (PVC). This type of plastic is found in some backpacks, folder covers, and raincoats. PVC may contain toxins that can be harmful to immune systems and is extremely difficult to recycle. In fact, of the 1.6 million tons of PVC discarded every year, the amount recycled is, at best, negligible. So check the product label for PVC disclosures or ask if what you're buying is made from PVC.

Plastic Rulers

Try to use plastic rulers made from 70 percent postconsumer recycled plastic. If every student in kindergarten through high school used one, we'd utilize 462 million inches of recycled plastic instead of 38.5 million feet of wood rulers or 7,291 miles of metal rulers.

Scissors

Try to use recycled stainless-steel scissors. If they have plastic handles, make sure it's at least 30 percent postconsumer plastic. Each year, steel recycling saves the energy equivalent of electrically powering about eighteen million homes for one year.

Tape Dispenser

Try to use a tape dispenser made of at least 50 percent postconsumer plastic. Plastic waste makes up 11 percent of landfills, and only 5 percent of it is recovered and used as recycled material.

Wastebaskets

Choose wastebaskets made from recycled steel. Steel is the most recycled material in the United States, and producing products from recycled steel requires 75 percent less energy than that required to manufacture products from iron ore.

Student Housing

Dorms

Live on-campus if you can. You'll cut down on commuting time, gasoline consumption, car maintenance, and pollution. There are eleven million college students, and 50 percent of those enrolled in state universities live off-campus. If half of these students could bike, walk, carpool, or take public transportation to school, more than two million commuter vehicles could be removed from the nation's busy streets and highways.

Laundry

Seek out energy-efficient (front-loader) laundry machines. Your clothes will wash and dry faster. There are about forty thousand coin laundries in the United States. If just one load in every Laundromat in the United States were washed by a front-loader washing machine instead of a top loader, we'd save a million gallons of water per day—as much as ten households use in a year.

FAITH HILL AND TIM McGRAW

"Our girls are very involved in recycling. Maggie, our eight-year-old, even wrote on the trash bin: "Please recycle here, thank you."

It all started when Zeny, a friend of ours, visited from San Francisco. She absolutely got us into shape on recycling. She was constantly reminding us that there was no other option. She'd tear apart boxes and even separate our garbage. When you get exposed to that level of teaching, it's something you never forget. And trust me, if anyone forgets, one of the girls is there to remind: Recycle! They're like minipolice. They separate their own glass bottles and cans. They even wash out their milk bottles and put things away. It's really amazing. If there is a carton on the counter, it doesn't stay there; it immediately gets put into the recycle bin. Recycling is also a great way to keep things clean!

You don't have to change the way you live to recycle. It really isn't all that big of a commitment. It's more about just being conscious of your waste. When you can see the difference recycling makes in your house, you can begin to imagine how big an impact it can have on the world.

And it all goes back to that simple little instruction written across our trash bin...."

work

Workin' for the Weekend and the World

THE BIG PICTURE

Maybe it's because we don't think of our office as our home, or we believe that if someone else is responsible for taking care of our paychecks, then they're responsible for our trash, too, but our offices have become skyscrapers of waste. They gorge on electricity, guzzle water, and expel toxins. They are beasts burdening our environment. The average office worker uses 10,000 sheets of copy paper each year. Across all U.S. businesses, the annual total is 21 million tons of copy paper, or more than 4 trillion sheets. About 400 billion photocopies are made each year, which means 750,000 copies are produced every minute. Besides paper, copies require ink. American businesses go through 15 million toner cartridges every year, enough to stretch from New York City to Zurich.

What drives all this is energy. Commercial buildings use 18 percent of all the energy in the country, and nearly one-quarter of that is used for lighting.

What's a shame is that a lot of office electricity is used to light offices when they are vacant or when there's sufficient natural light to go without lamps or overhead lighting.

In addition to sapping energy, office buildings are responsible for more than 10 percent of all the water used in the United States. Last we checked, most people aren't showering, watering lawns, doing dishes, or laundering clothes at the office. Workers are mostly flushing and washing their hands . . . at least we hope they are.

What we do know is that workers drive an average of ten thousand miles a year. We call it commuting. In doing so, they use 67.5 billion gallons of gasoline. This would be bad enough if they all stayed put at their desks. But one-third of all workers leave the office to buy food, and they spend most of their lunch hour getting it. The waste from lunch alone amounts to enough disposable cups and plastic utensils to more than circle the equator every workday!

Food waste is another problem. Ten percent of all the waste produced by an office is food. Imagine that multiplied by every business in the country. That's an awful lot of ketchup, mustard, and salt and pepper packets.

But the office supply room contributes the most to the office waste problem, with tons of paper, pens, paper clips, and rubber bands being needlessly tossed out.

To be sure, most of us aren't in charge of our office policies. We can't order more environmentally friendly supplies, adjust the thermostat for the whole building we work in, or mind the trash for recycling. But there are some things we can do individually to help work for the environment at the office.

Keeping all that in mind, we've created the "Simple Steps" to be just that. Taking into account all the points of the Big Picture, they give you the biggest impact with the least amount of effort.

The Simple Steps

1. **Double-side your copies.** Whether printing or copying, use both sides of a piece of paper. If just one in four office workers made all of their copies double-sided, the annual savings would equal 130 billion sheets of paper—a stack thicker than the diameter of the earth!

2. **Carpool.** If the average commuter carpooled every day, he or she would save five hundred gallons of gasoline, and 550 pounds of poisonous exhaust emissions every year. Commuters sharing a ride to work would be the equivalent of taking 67.5 million cars off the road—four times the number of new cars sold in the United States per year.

3. **Use a ceramic mug for your coffee.** Americans use more than fourteen billion paper cups every year, enough to circle the world fifty-five times. The Styrofoam kind will stay on the planet for nine generations, enough time for your great-great-great-great-great-great-great-great-grandkids to be born.

THE LITTLE THINGS

Getting There

Car

Keeping your tires fully inflated could improve your gas mileage by around 3 percent. (It also makes your tires last longer.) The average American, who drives twelve thousand miles per year, could save about 16 gallons of gasoline annually (assuming 25 mpg) just by maintaining his or her tires at the proper pressure. Across all U.S. households, the gasoline savings could total 1.6 billion gallons—approximately the total volume of ice cream produced in the United States each year.

Public Transportation

Try to take public transportation. If all Americans who take transit to work drove alone, they would fill a nine-lane freeway from Boston to Los Angeles. Fewer cars on the road also significantly reduces commuting time. People spend an average of thirty-six hours—nearly five full workdays—in traffic delays per year.

Telecommute

Join the forty-four million people who work from home at least part-time. Telecommuting prevents more than thirty-five billion vehicle miles traveled per year and saves almost two billion gallons of gasoline.

Walk

Walk and your commute is free. People who live within two miles of their office still spend $384 a year to drive back and forth. If just twenty people in every state did it, we'd save more than sixty-four thousand pounds of harmful chemicals from being released into the air—roughly the amount of toxic air pollutants emitted by industrial facilities within Washington, D.C., each year.

In the Break Room

Coffeemaker

Mind the amount of water you use when brewing. Making coffee uses about a third of the tap water consumed in most of North America and Europe. If every worker cut back on water fill by one cup, we'd save almost ten million gallons per day. Over the course of a year, this would save enough water to provide two gallons to the 1.2 billion people on the planet who don't have access to safe water at all.

Stirrers

Don't use disposable stirrers. Just pour in your sugar and milk first then add coffee. Each year, Americans throw away 138 billion straws and stirrers, enough to make a giant straw statue—twenty times taller than the Statue of Liberty!

Sugar/Sweeteners

Use loose containers rather than individual packets. When you use individual packets of sugar, you're using about as much packaging as the sweetener in it.

Meal Breaks

Cafeteria

Use silverware and plates, not plasticware, in the cafeteria if you have a choice. Even one office worker using just 1 plastic knife per day could add up to 250 a year. If every other worker used just 1 a day, it would amount to 15 billion plastic knives a year, enough to create a plastic blade 1.5 million miles long.

Food Storage

Choose glass or ceramic containers that can be reused. They're healthier than plastic, and you'll reduce the waste generated. Four out of five office workers share food brought in by fellow employees. Using glass or ceramic for this food reduces the possibility that you or your co-workers will be exposed to harmful seepage from plastic containers. You'll also avoid creating additional waste from disposable trays, plates, and containers.

Litter

Dispose of waste properly. Ninety-four percent of people identify litter as a major environmental problem. The biggest sources of litter are cigarette butts, bottles and cans (including tops and ring pulls), candy wrappers, and fast-food packaging. More than two billion pounds of cigarette butts are discarded worldwide—about two pounds for every person in China.

Lunch

Bring your lunch from home if you can. A disposable lunch creates between four and eight ounces of garbage every day. That can add up to as much as one hundred pounds per year! Bringing lunch from home could result in the U.S. workforce saving more than ten billion pounds of trash—equal to the weight of the Great Pyramid in Egypt.

Paper Napkins

Try to use fewer paper napkins. Each American consumes an average of 2,200 two-ply napkins per year, or just over 6 napkins per day. If each worker used just 1 fewer napkin per day, it would save about 150 million of them from the trash—enough to provide a napkin to every person who eats a hot dog on July 4.

Takeout

Request less packaging when you order your food to go. More than a third of office workers order in or carry out from a restaurant. If the takeout is just for you, tell the restaurant you need utensils only for one. If every worker did this, we could save twenty-five million plastic forks, knives, and chopsticks per day—enough utensils for three square meals a day for everyone in New York City.

In the Supply Room

Copier

Using the "standby" button on your copier will lighten your energy load by 70 percent. It costs about $50 million to power the nation's copiers annually. Cut that by 70 percent and save $35 million and enough energy to provide a month's worth of electricity to more than one hundred thousand homes.

Correction Fluid

Try using a correction pen as opposed to bottled correction liquid. It won't dry out as fast, and you'll likely use less. Also, make sure the correction fluid you use is water based. If every office assistant used one less bottle of correction fluid per year, the savings could coat the White House.

Envelopes

Use postconsumer recycled envelopes. Just seventeen workers in an office go through a ton of paper, including envelopes and copy paper, each year. If offices used recycled envelopes instead of envelopes made from virgin paper, each of these seventeen workers would save enough paper materials to mail a letter to every one of their ten thousand closest friends.

Fax Machines

Avoid a cover page when possible and you'll save paper on both ends of the transmission. Seventeen million trees per year are cut down to supply fax paper for the United States.

Labels

Try not to use them, or use those that have recycled content. Some labels make it impossible to recycle the paper, envelopes, or other materials to which they might be stuck. Instead, try printing directly onto envelopes and packages.

Packaging/Shipping

You don't have to put a box inside a shipping box or an envelope inside a letter pack. Over one billion overnight shipping boxes and envelopes are used each year. If just 1 percent of those boxes were saved, it would be enough packaging for two holiday gifts for every child under the age of five in the United States.

Paper
Recycle, and try to use recycled paper. American businesses use over twenty-one million tons of paper annually. If half of this were recycled paper, a forest larger than the state of Florida could be saved every year.

Paper Clips
Reuse your paper clips. Enough paper clips are produced to hand every person in the country at least three. If one out of every four workers reused their paper clips, it would save more than $1 million.

Pens
Try to use refillable pens, pencils, and markers. Disposable plastic pens aren't recyclable, nor are they biodegradable. Throw one away, and it will still be in a landfill fifty thousand years from now.

Postage Meters
Try printing online stamps instead of using a postage meter. You'll save on equipment, maintenance, and money. Besides, postage meters use more ink than printing stamps online—an additional $27 million worth of ink for U.S. businesses per month. When ink dissolves from products at a landfill, it can release harmful chemicals into the ground.

Printers
Print double-sided pages, and use an inkjet if you can. Laser printers use three hundred watts of electricity, while inkjets use only ten. Workers can save the equivalent of 5 percent of all home electricity usage in the United States, or the amount of energy contained in four lightning bolts, by using an inkjet printer instead of a laser printer. And of course, don't forget to recycle your ink cartridge.

Recycle

Recycle at your desk and in the office supply room. Just by recycling paper, offices can reduce by 50 percent the waste they send to landfills. This is a savings of thirty-three million tons—enough to save 561 million trees.

Rubber Bands

Avoid using rubber bands if you can. About three-quarters of rubber bands are synthetic, made from crude oil. When these are incinerated at the dump, significant health effects can result. In North America, 2.2 million metric tons of synthetic rubbers are used per year. This could make almost a quarter of a million rubber band balls as big as the world's largest ball of twine (in Cawker City, Kansas).

Staples

Use an eco-stapler, which doesn't use metal staples, for tasks that require binding five pages or less. Some 643,000 metric tons of staples are produced annually in the United States. If one-third of the documents that are stapled could be bound without staples, we could keep nearly a trillion staples out of the trash each year.

At Your Desk

Computers

Activate the power management function, or sleep mode, on your monitors and CPU boxes. If just ten employees did it, they'd save nearly $500 in energy costs per year.

Cooling

Try to use space fans rather than air-conditioning. Air-conditioning accounts for the second highest use of electricity (approximately 15 percent of total consumption) in commercial buildings. Being more energy efficient with cooling during peak summer months in just the western region of the United States could save enough electricity to power three hundred thousand homes for a whole year.

E-Mail

More than two hours of the average office worker's time is used per day sending e-mails and surfing the Internet. Internet data servers use as much energy in the United States as is used by all U.S. TVs combined.

Heating

Try to keep your office at a constant temperature, between sixty-nine and seventy-three degrees Fahrenheit. About half of all the energy used in commercial buildings is for space heating and cooling. Businesses can cut their usage costs by one-third just by being more energy efficient and can reduce air pollution equivalent to the exhaust from forty million cars because of all the carbon emissions saved from using less energy.

Lighting

Turn off your office lights if natural light from the sun is available. You'll get less eye fatigue due to glare. Seventeen percent of the energy used for lighting offices is wasted when offices are left vacant or lights are unnecessarily turned on in a sunlit room. That wasted energy is enough to drive a car to Jupiter.

Virtual Meetings

Save time and money by teleconferencing. Avoid the average business trip by airplane and you'll save enough energy to conduct seven thousand hours of videoconferences!

" When I was a young girl growing up in Nutley, New Jersey, the environment wasn't yet a cause for concern. Instead, economy was, at least for my parents, who had the challenging task of providing for six children. Every day my mother cooked simple yet delicious meals using seasonal produce and meat, which were always a better bargain. My father, on the other hand, was passionate about gardening, and the fruits of his labor—greens in the spring, tomatoes in the summer, squash in the fall— always livened up our dinner table. Lamps were only illuminated when necessary, heat was used in moderation, and as a result we learned to be frugal with resources.

Looking back on those years, I have realized that my family's routines followed many of the "green living" guidelines that books like this one are now discussing. A generation later, the environment is now a subject on everyone's minds, including mine. Here are some of the eco-friendly practices I've put into use on my farm in Bedford, New York. Of these, some are recent technological advances, such as compact-fluorescent light bulbs and alternative fuels. Many of the rest are the habits and lessons that I learned from my parents decades ago.

To name a few, gardening has always been a love of mine, and at my Bedford farm we follow organic principles in the vegetable and cutting gardens, as well as in the greenhouse. I also maintain a giant compost heap, which turns produce scraps, yard trimmings, and horse manure into valuable fertilizer. In addition to recycling conventional things such as cans and bottles, I use salvaged building materials in various projects around the farm. Just recently we constructed new chicken coops using slate shingles from an old Vermont farmhouse to create the roofs and wood boards cut from the farm for the floor. Providing homes for wild birds is also important to me: We hang owl boxes around the property to give them a place to nest. Bluebirds have quickly established colonies in homes we provided. Barn swallows and their mud nests are welcomed as natural "mosquito eaters."

In my home, good insulation and an efficient heating system are two of the easiest ways to reduce energy costs, which is good for me and the environment. I have always used storm windows in the wintertime, which help reduce air flow in and out of the house. I also have an efficient, under-floor radiant heating system, which requires lower water temperatures than conventional radiators and concentrates heat at a lower level in the room, rather than at the ceiling. As a result, I set the thermostat lower than most in the wintertime—at 64°F, instead of 72°F. I buy Energy Star appliances and have switched the light bulbs in my house to energy-efficient compact-fluorescent ones. I also use small, quiet electric fans to move the air in the hot weather, allowing me to use only minimal air-conditioning.

Here are five things you can do:

1) Buy five-gallon jugs of water and refill bottles for daily consumption.
2) Turn off lights when you leave a room.
3) Turn off or lower heat when you leave for work.
4) Use a down comforter instead of running the heat.
5) Use reusable rags instead of paper towels.

Over the coming years, there will be new ways to live in better harmony with the environment. In the meantime, my latest project is to use alternative, ethanol-based fuels instead of gasoline in some of the cars and farm vehicles. Every little bit helps. My mother would certainly agree and my daughter, too. "

shopping

Good Things Come in Small Packages, Especially When They're Not Wrapped

THE BIG PICTURE

The United States is the world's top consumer nation. Americans spend about four times more per person than any other country. And we do it largely by shopping. We shop, on average, every day for about twenty-four minutes, spending a total of about $4 trillion per year—on everything from waffles to Wiffle balls.

Every time we hit the mall, we spend an average of $113. We want lots of stuff and create huge demand for consumer products of all types. A new car is made every second, 2.3 million shoes are purchased every day, and 2.6 billion toys are bought every year.

The psychology of shopping is embedded in our brains: more, more, more. The mentality fills the closets and the ego but doesn't take into account the other side of the shopping equation—where does all that stuff go?

Each of us produces about 4.54 pounds of trash every day through our consumption and disposal habits, amounting to 1,657 pounds per person per year. As a nation, that adds up to about 500 billion pounds annually.

The disposal burden is enormous—so much so that if you look at North America from space, the highest point on the eastern seaboard is a landfill.

How does a pile get that high? Consider that every month, one hundred thousand CDs are tossed; or that fifty million pounds of toothbrushes are scattered throughout the country's landfills every year. Soon, you get the picture. And this truly is a big picture.

We use tons of materials, water, and energy to make the things we buy—only to discard them later; it's a disposable society.

With 6.6 billion people on the planet (and growing), all eventually apt to buy something and throw it away, shopping poses a real hazard. Think of it this way: There is more man-made stuff than people on the planet. The average family around the world has no fewer than 127 items in their home. In the United States, the number of objects in an average family home can amount to 10,000.

So how does all that stuff come to exist? It's manufactured. The manufacturing industry alone sucks one-third of the energy and 13 percent of the water supply in the United States, never mind all the additional waste (7.6 billion tons of it) that's produced before the products even reach our hands.

And then we toss it all back onto the planet. More than 1.5 billion tons of household solid waste is produced every year around the world. That's equivalent to almost three times the total weight of every person alive! Disposal is such a big issue that the United States often ships its waste to other countries. More than half of the electronics we import end up being exported to third world countries as waste. The other half continues to pile up right here at home.

Keeping all that in mind, we've created the "Simple Steps" to be just that. Taking into account all the points of the Big Picture, they give you the biggest impact with the least amount of effort.

The Simple Steps

1. **Try to buy products with minimal to no packaging.** If just one out of ten products you bought had little or no packaging, it would eliminate more than fifty pounds of waste per household per year. This small reduction could also save you at least $30 annually, as $1 of every $11 that you spend at the supermarket pays for the packaging of the products you buy. If every household did this, 5.5 billion fewer pounds of waste would enter landfills. This is enough garbage to cover all of New York City's Central Park to a depth of twenty-seven feet.

2. **If you're asked, "paper or plastic?" at checkout, choose paper.** While neither is an ideal choice—it's best to sack your groceries in reusable cloth or canvas bags—grocery baggers usually fill paper bags with more items than they do plastic bags, and paper bags can be easily reused. Moreover, paper bags have a better chance of being recycled.

3. **Switch to bathroom tissue made from 100 percent recycled paper.** If every household replaced just a single twelve-roll pack of regular bathroom tissue with a recycled variety, it would save almost five million trees and enough paper waste to fill seventeen thousand garbage trucks.

THE LITTLE THINGS

Groceries

Bread—Dinner

If possible, buy your dinner breads fresh from the grocery store bakery. You can recycle the paper wrapper and save on energy used for freezing and transporting the shelf-bought brands. If every U.S. household served fresh-baked bread instead of packaged rolls for Thanksgiving dinner, the energy conserved could fly more than twenty-three thousand early colonists from England to Plymouth Rock.

Bread—Sliced

If you buy sliced bread from the bread aisle, try to find loaves that are packaged in only a single wrapper. Double-wrapped loaves contain at least 20 percent more plastic packaging—per gram of bread. The waste generated by this additional wrapper across all households in the United States and Canada would weigh nearly sixty thousand pounds— or the total weight of all the food you will ever eat in your lifetime.

Bulk

Consider buying items in bulk. You will pay up to 50 percent less and significantly reduce the amount of energy needed to transport all that extra packaging waste to landfills and recycling facilities. If by buying in bulk every U.S. household generated 10 percent less packaging waste, the volume of diesel fuel saved by garbage trucks annually would be enough to take a busload of schoolchildren on a field trip to the moon and back every day of the school year.

Canned Goods

If you're planning to purchase several cans of the same product, look to see if a larger can is available. If you buy a 28-ounce can of stewed tomatoes instead of two 14.5-ounce cans, you'll not only save up to 50 percent on the price, but you'll also reduce waste and conserve resources. If every month each U.S. household substituted a larger can for two smaller ones, the annual savings in steel could build an Eiffel Tower on each of the six other continents.

Cheese

Buy block cheese instead of presliced individually wrapped servings. The energy used to make the plastic wrappers for slices of American cheese amounts to the equivalent of more than 13.8 million gallons of gasoline per year—enough for the entire population of Milwaukee to carpool out west to visit the happy cows of California.

Coffee

When you buy ground or whole-bean coffee, look for varieties with organic, Fair Trade, Bird Friendly, or Rainforest Alliance certification seals. These labels represent coffee farms that practice sustainable agriculture to preserve or restore rain forest ecosystems. Just one household switching to certified coffee for a year is enough to protect 9,200 square feet of rain forest. If everyone in Seattle switched to certified coffees, a rain forest area the size of that city could be saved every year.

Farmer's Market vs. Supermarket

Try doing some of your shopping at a local farmer's market. And if you can, walk or bike there. Of the total energy used in the United States per year, 4 percent is used to produce food, and between 10 and 13 percent is used to transport it. On average, U.S. supermarket food travels 1,500 to 2,500 miles before it reaches the family table. Buying local food can reduce the amount of petroleum consumed to transport your dinner by as much as 95 percent.

Fish—Farmed vs. Wild

Choose sustainably harvested wild fish as opposed to farmed varieties. Farmed fish tend to have higher levels of heavy metals and are considered threats to endangered populations of wild fish species. Also, because farmed fish live in extremely close quarters, they generate a lot of waste. The volume of fish feces that enters the tide from the average fish farm is equal to a town of sixty-five thousand people releasing their untreated raw sewage directly into the ocean.

Fish—Fresh vs. Canned

Consider purchasing fresh fish instead of canned fish. You will reduce the amount of resources wasted in the canning process and might even save money. For every ten pounds of canned fish produced, twenty gallons of water and more than half a pound of edible fish are wasted. Given that a six-ounce can of fish generally contains only about four ounces of meat, the price for canned fish ($4 to $8 per pound) is actually comparable to that of some fresh fish varieties. If each of the eighty-eight million U.S. households that buy canned tuna replaced just one six-ounce can with a six-ounce purchase of fresh fish, the water and fish saved could fill a seventy-foot-high aquarium spanning two soccer fields with more than twelve thousand one-hundred-pound yellowfin tuna.

Fruit

Try to limit purchases of canned fruit, and substitute fresh fruit whenever possible. The process involved with canning fruit is at least ten times more energy intensive than picking fresh fruit. If every U.S. household replaced just one pound of canned or jarred fruit with one pound of fresh fruit during each of the three summer months, the total energy saved could operate the kitchen appliances of over twenty-one thousand households for an entire year.

Meat

If you have the option, choose your meat at the butcher counter and purchase only as much as you know you'll use. You'll reduce food waste, save money, and conserve resources. The average person wastes over twenty-two pounds of edible store-bought meat each year. Given that it takes five pounds of grain and 2,500 gallons of water to make one pound of beef, that's more than one hundred pounds of wasted grain and 55,000 gallons of wasted water per person! If all households decreased their beef purchases by just one pound per year, 250 billion gallons of water would be saved. It would take five days for this amount of water to pour over Niagara Falls.

Milk

Buy a single gallon jug instead of purchasing multiple smaller containers. On a volume basis, it takes less energy to produce the bigger containers and generates less waste. The average household buying sixty-three gallons of milk per year (including flavored) could run its refrigerator for thirty-six hours with the energy saved by purchasing bigger containers.

Organic

You can lower your exposure to pesticides by 90 percent just by choosing organic varieties of certain fruits and vegetables. If just 1 percent of the nation's farmlands converted to organic (nonchemical) agricultural systems, it would remove twenty-six million pounds of pesticides per year from the food we eat and from the environment. If you buy organic, you'll encourage this type of farming.

Paper Bags

Reuse your paper bags from the grocery store as trash liners. By reusing a paper grocery sack three times before recycling or retiring it as a trash can liner, the average U.S. household could reduce the production of virgin-forest-derived paper by fifty-five pounds per year. If just 5 percent of U.S. households adopted this habit, the effect in terms of trees saved per year would be a mature forest the size of Manhattan. After thirteen years, the forest would cover all of New York City.

Paper Towels

If you can, select paper towel rolls with smaller-size sheets in order to extend the life of each roll. (Check the package label for sheet sizes.)

A decrease in U.S. household consumption of just three rolls per year would save 120,000 tons of waste and $4.1 million in landfill dumping fees.

Plastic Bags

Use fewer plastic bags. U.S. households dispose of nearly one hundred billion plastic bags annually, millions of which end up littering the environment and harming endangered marine animals. By reducing plastic bag consumption by just two bags per week, you'll throw away at least one hundred fewer bags per year. If tied together handle to handle, these plastic bags would make a rope long enough to wrap around the earth more than 126 times.

Poultry

When you buy poultry, try to buy only as much as you think you'll need. On average, each American throws away about twelve pounds of uneaten poultry per year. If over the course of a year each household purchased just one less pound of chicken, the total water saved by not having to package and produce it would be sixty-six billion gallons—more than all of the residents of California use in a week.

Soy

Consider buying soy food products. Growing soybeans doesn't require nearly the amount of water that's needed to raise animals. A household that replaces one pound of beef with one pound of soy per month will conserve twenty thousand gallons of water per year. If just 20 percent of households in the United States and Canada substituted four ounces of beef for four ounces of soy per week, the annual water savings would be enough to provide ten gallons of drinking water to every person in the world.

Trash Bags

If you need to purchase trash liner bags, look for a brand with 100 percent postconsumer recycled content. Producing trash bags from recycled plastic requires less energy than manufacturing those same bags from virgin plastic. If just one in ten U.S. households began purchasing trash bags made from 100 percent recycled materials, the annual energy savings could meet the heating needs of four thousand households in Fargo, North Dakota, for the entire year.

Vegetables

If you have the option, choose fresh vegetables over canned or frozen ones. Freezing and canning fresh vegetables in the United States uses about three billion kilowatt-hours of energy per year, which is enough power to light every light bulb in the state of New York for three years. When in season, fresh vegetables can also cost less than canned or frozen varieties.

Clothing

Dyes

The process of dyeing fabric generates the largest proportion of wastewater produced by the textile industry. So buy clothes with "natural" colors. If most Americans chose one pair of pants that weren't dyed—it would save enough dye to cover the entire city of Chicago with an inch of colorful liquid.

Fabric

Consider buying clothes made from organic cotton. The purchase of one T-shirt and a pair of jeans made from 100 percent organic cotton eliminates at least 150 grams of fertilizers, pesticides, and herbicides from the environment. If one out of every five Americans purchased a

100 percent organic T-shirt instead of one made from conventionally grown U.S. cotton, nearly fifty thousand tons of agrochemicals would be prevented from polluting U.S. freshwater bodies, ecosystems, and wardrobes.

Fur

You can add fossil fuel consumption to the list of reasons not to buy real fur. Although synthetic fur is made from petroleum products, it takes only one-third of a gallon of oil to produce a faux fur jacket, while it takes twenty-two gallons of oil to produce the energy needed to make one from real fur. If just 10 percent of the three million real fur garments sold in the United States each year were replaced by an alternative nonfur garment, an average of five million gallons of oil and five million animals could be saved.

Secondhand Clothing

Give secondhand clothing a chance. The average American purchases forty-eight articles of new clothing per year. If just one of those articles were purchased from a secondhand store, the energy equivalent of more than half a gallon of gasoline could be saved, because of all the energy used to manufacture and transport new clothes. If one in every ten Americans substituted his or her next purchase of one new garment with a vintage one, the energy saved could fly every resident of Hollywood to New York City for Fashion Week.

Shoes

You can reduce the size of your footprint on the environment by purchasing shoes made from recycled materials. Look for soles made from postconsumer tire rubber, insoles made from foam cushions, or canvas made from old jackets or jeans. Your new footprint could represent the reuse and recycling of almost anything from soda bottles, foam cups,

milk jugs, cardboard, and magazines to denim, coffee filters, file folders, cork, blankets, and burlap sacks. If every American household purchased one pair of shoes made from recycled materials, the savings
could total more than two hundred million pounds of waste diverted
from landfills.

Health

Homeopathic vs. Manufactured Pharmaceuticals
Consider using homeopathic medicines instead of over-the-counter or
prescription pharmaceuticals to treat medical conditions. The process of
manufacturing synthetic drugs emits more than 177 million pounds of
untreated pollutants into air, water, and soil resources each year. If just
5 percent of the population could find a homeopathic remedy for half
their medication needs, fewer pollutants—4.4 million pounds' worth—
would make it into the water system.

Prescription Medication
Fill only those prescriptions you're sure you will use, and never flush unused or expired prescriptions down the toilet or drain. Pharmaceuticals
in wastewater have been found to damage plants, fish, and animals.
Because so much medicine is wasted, if the average patient over age
sixty-five who fills twenty-four prescriptions annually purchased only
those drugs that would be fully consumed, he or she could save $70 per
year at the pharmacy. From all patients, the amount of medication
saved could fill a giant forty-five-foot-tall medicine bottle each year.

Vitamins
You can save money and packaging waste if you buy a multivitamin
rather than separate bottles of individual vitamins. The average American
vitamin user spends over $100 each year on vitamins and supplements. If
one-quarter of vitamin consumers reduced their purchases by just one

bottle per year, the estimated total savings would be $592 million and 103 stacks of plastic bottles, each tall enough to reach the top of the ozone layer.

Pets

Collars/Leashes

Try purchasing a pet leash or collar that is made from organic canvas materials instead of nylon. Nylon production emits nitrous oxide—a type of greenhouse gas associated with global warming. If every dog in the United States eventually received a replacement leash made of organic fibers instead of nylon, it would prevent the release of as much greenhouse gases as 250,000 households produce each year.

Fish Tanks

When you clean your fish tank, remove only one-third to one-half of the water and use it as a nutrient-rich solution for house and outdoor plants. You'll conserve water and eliminate the need for chemical fertilizers. If every fish owner adopted this habit, the freshwater saved annually would be enough to fill two twenty-four-ounce bottles for each of the 1.2 billion people in the world without access to safe drinking water.

Pet Beds

The next time your canine or feline friend needs a new bed, look for one that is filled with recycled fiber. If just one in every twenty dog owners purchased a bed made from recycled materials, the fiber savings would total nearly 3,200 tons and fill four hundred garbage trucks.

Pet Food

Consider a vegetarian diet for your pets, or at least consider feeding them less meat, poultry, and fish. It takes less energy to manufacture vegetarian pet food because of the processing involved. If every dog in the United States ate vegetarian one day per month, the energy savings per year would be the equivalent of 190 million gallons of gasoline—enough to drive every dog in the United States to an annual dog show seventy-five miles away.

Pet Toys
Choose pet toys made from recycled materials. If all pet toys purchased each year boasted 100 percent recycled content, the virgin materials saved could make a Frisbee nearly 2.5 miles in diameter.

Pet Treats
If you buy pet treats with no packaging or in packaging that can be recycled, you will prevent a pound or more of plastic from entering landfills each year. If 10 percent of all dog and cat owners purchased pet treats in recyclable packaging, more than fifty-eight thousand cubic yards of waste would be eliminated annually. If this waste were packed into a standard three-acre dog park, it would tower more than twelve feet high.

Lawn and Garden

Fertilizers
The average home with four thousand square feet of lawn can reduce fertilizer requirements by 25 percent, or about three pounds per year, by leaving grass clippings on the lawn after mowing. It takes more than a gallon of diesel fuel to make three pounds of fertilizer. If home owners "grass-cycled" and reduced their fertilizer use by just 25 percent, it would save 1.3 billion pounds of chemical fertilizers and more diesel fuel than Amtrak uses in six years.

Floral Arrangements
If you buy fresh flowers, seek out varieties that are grown locally and organically. The application of toxins and chemicals used to grow fresh

flowers can pollute water systems. Buy organically grown varieties and you help reduce the amount of pesticides used. If all roses purchased for Valentine's Day were organically grown, it would prevent the use of 22,700 pounds of pesticides—equivalent to the weight of a giant chocolate Hershey's Kiss more than ten feet tall.

Flowers

Look for outdoor flowers and shrubs with low water requirements and you could save up to 550 gallons of water per year. If just one in every one hundred households chose drought-tolerant species of flowers for the next replanting, nearly 600 million gallons of water could be conserved—enough to provide New York City its residential water supply for an entire day.

Outdoor Furniture

Look for outdoor patio furniture made from recycled materials instead of from wood or metal. One bench made from recycled materials can prevent the equivalent of two thousand plastic bottles from entering landfills.

Sprinklers

Buy adjustable sprinkler heads to maximize watering efficiency and water coverage on your lawn. If a half-circle sprinkler head could be reduced to about one-third of a circle without losing water coverage, you could decrease your watering time and save about two hundred gallons of water per year.

Kids

Baby Body Wash

There is no need to buy expensive body washes when mild soap and warm water will work perfectly well for bathing your baby. If you purchase paper-wrapped soap instead of plastic bottles of body wash, you will save on money and packaging. If every baby born this year were bathed with a bar of baby soap instead of a bottle of body wash, the plastic packaging saved would weigh more than two hundred thousand pounds—enough to make a baby bathtub that would cover more than four acres.

Baby Food

Buy organic baby food in reusable glass jars or recyclable paper boxes. By selecting reusable glass jars or recyclable boxes over plastic containers, you will reduce the amount of waste sent to landfills. If every year just 1 percent of baby food jars (six jars per baby) were saved and reused for storage, reheating, crafts, and the like, the weight saved in glass would tip the scales at 680,000 pounds, about as much as a Boeing 747.

Baby Lotion

If you buy baby lotion, aim for a container that can be reused and eventually recycled. If you avoid the nonrecyclable plastic squeeze tube, you will prevent about one ounce of packaging from being wasted. If just 10 percent of the babies born this year used lotion in a recyclable or reusable container, roughly twenty thousand pounds of plastic could be saved from landfills.

Baby Shampoo

When there are various sizes of baby shampoo to choose from, you'll save money and resources by selecting the largest size available. If you choose a fifteen-ounce bottle of baby shampoo instead of two seven-ounce bottles, you could save more than $1.50 per purchase, about twenty-two grams of plastic, and get an extra ounce of shampoo for free. Across 10 percent of babies born this year, the estimated savings from purchasing one large bottle of shampoo instead of two smaller bottles would be over $600,000 and twenty thousand pounds of plastic.

Baby Wipes

Avoid buying baby wipes in hard plastic packaging if you already have a reusable container at home. If you choose refill packs instead, you will reduce the packaging you buy by about 1.5 pounds or more per month. If all babies born this year used refill packs instead of hard plastic containers, the manufacturing energy saved could wash and dry one load of laundry for every U.S. household.

Batteries

Consider purchasing rechargeable batteries for your child's battery-operated toys. Four rechargeable AA alkaline batteries can reduce the need to buy and dispose of roughly one hundred conventional batteries—an eventual savings of approximately $40 and eight pounds of hazardous waste. If 10 percent of children under twelve used rechargeable batteries for dolls, action figures, remote-control cars, and so forth, an estimated thirty-eight million single-use batteries could be saved from disposal. The energy from these batteries could power an electric car to circle the earth seventeen times.

Cloth vs. Disposable Diapers

Try using cloth diapers (preferably from organic cotton) instead of disposable diapers. Over the course of eight thousand diaper changes, your baby will generate three thousand fewer pounds of landfill waste. If cloth diapers were used by just an additional 1 percent of parents, the reduction in waste would be as if 14,200 households completely stopped producing garbage for an entire year.

Cotton Swabs

Choose double-tipped cotton swabs (preferably organic) that are connected with spindles made from tightly rolled paper over those made from plastic. Paperboard spindles are potentially biodegradable and use renewable resources, whereas plastic spindles are made from petroleum and will not biodegrade. Across 10 percent of U.S. households, the petroleum energy saved per year would be equivalent to over 150,000 gallons of gasoline.

Laundry Soap

Look for baby laundry liquids that contain vegetable-based cleaners instead of those that are petroleum based. They're gentler on your baby and won't contribute to the depletion of fossil fuels. If all babies born this year had their clothes laundered in a vegetable-based detergent, the petroleum saved would equal 1.5 million gallons of gasoline, or the equivalent amount of energy to wash about ten million loads of laundry.

Strollers

Try to avoid buying carriages that will accommodate your baby only for the first few months after birth. If you buy a single sturdy adjustable stroller that will fit the needs and size of your baby as he or she grows, you will save at least $150 as well as the environmental resources used to produce an additional stroller for your child. If every child born in the United States today received a single stroller that could work throughout toddlerhood, the money saved could run 25,625 night-lights for fifty years.

Toy Manufacturers

Try frequenting shops that sell locally made toys. Of all toys purchased in the United States, 80 percent are made overseas, and 71 percent are made in China, where environmental laws are weak. If you support locally produced goods, you could reduce the pollution and fuel costs associated with shipping products across the Pacific Ocean.

Toy Packaging

Try to buy toys with the least amount of packaging possible. Americans buy 3.6 billion toys per year, and in some cases the packaging volume for a single toy can be more than ten times the size of the toy itself. If all of the packaging sold with action figures each year were combined to make one giant package, it could hold an action figure that was more than 4,700 miles tall!

Toys

Avoid buying plastic teething rings, rattles, bath toys, plastic books, squeeze toys, or any other plastic product that your child may put in his or her mouth. If you choose baby toys that are made from natural products such as sustainable wood and organic cotton, you'll reduce your baby's exposure to potentially harmful toxins as well as conserve the energy associated with the manufacturing of plastics. If all babies born in the United States this year were given natural alternatives to plastic teething toys, the energy conserved could power a thirty-two-inch television to run nonstop reruns of *Sesame Street* for fifteen straight years.

Toys—Plastic

Look for toys made from materials other than plastic. Many plastic toys (including dolls and action figures) are made of PVC and contain toxins known as phthalates that are potentially harmful to both the environment and children's health. If every child under twelve received just one alternative-to-plastic birthday gift this year, not only could an estimated twenty-five million pounds of plastic toys be diverted from landfills, but the total energy savings could bake thirty-one million birthday cakes.

Toys—Wood

Buy wooden alternatives to plastic toys whenever possible. Nontoxic solid wood toys are potentially not only better for the health of your child, but they use renewable resources (as opposed to plastics, which are petroleum based). If every child under six today received a quality wooden version of a plastic toy that could be passed down to a younger child next year, the result could be a decrease of some seventeen million pounds of landfilled plastic for each year the toy is reused.

Holidays

Candles

Because paraffin wax candles are made from petroleum and release the equivalent of diesel exhaust when burned, you can save fossil fuel resources, improve your indoor air quality, and reduce your exposure to carcinogens by choosing 100 percent beeswax or soy candles. These candles are not only made from renewable resources, but burn 90 percent cleaner and at least 50 percent longer than conventional paraffin candles. The crude oil used to make just one sixteen-ounce paraffin candle contains enough energy to power a sixty-watt light bulb for one hundred hours. If just one in a hundred households replaced an eight-ounce petroleum-based candle with a soy or beeswax candle, the energy saved could keep the Christmas tree in Rockefeller Center lit 24/7 from Thanksgiving until the Fourth of July.

Christmas Trees

If you're planning to purchase a tree this Christmas, the greenest choice is a living tree that can be reused or replanted. If this is not an option, natural cut trees are preferable to artificial varieties. Although artificial trees are potentially endlessly reusable, they are usually made from non-renewable PVC plastic, contain trace amounts of lead, and tend to be discarded after only six holiday seasons. Real Christmas trees (especially organic ones) provide environmental benefits, as they grow and can be recycled easily after the new year. If just 10 percent of households planning to purchase a new artificial tree this year purchased a natural one instead, forty-four million pounds of nonbiodegradable materials could be conserved and diverted from landfills.

Decorations

If you're planning to buy holiday decorations this year, consider a decor of seasonal plants (poinsettia, holly, pinecones), decorations that can be reused or donated, or vintage items from an antiques shop. Two-thirds of households buy new Christmas decorations each year and spend over $7.5 billion. If these households diverted just $6 of their decorating budget to reusable items, the money saved could pay to heat 5.9 million New England homes for every hour between Christmas and New Year's Day.

Gift Giving

Gift cards, concert tickets, restaurant certificates, and movie vouchers can be great alternatives to heavily packaged and wrapped holiday presents. If you buy these items online, you'll not only save between five and ten pounds of packaging waste, you'll also reduce the time, stress, and energy associated with traffic, crowds, and long checkout lines. If 50 percent of households replaced just two packaged presents with gifts that could slide inside an envelope, fifty million pounds or more of waste could be saved.

Greeting Cards

Purchase greeting cards made from recycled or tree-free materials. Americans send two billion holiday cards each year, so just a 1 percent reduction could save fifteen thousand trees.

Holiday Lights

When you replace your holiday lights, you can save significant money and energy by choosing LED (light-emitting diode) types. Three one-hundred-light strands of LED bulbs running for five hours every day between Thanksgiving and New Year's will use on average only 3 kilowatt-hours—an energy cost of only thirty cents. For the same period of time, large incandescent bulbs will spin your meter at a rate of 472 kilowatt-hours and to the tune of nearly $60. With a one-hundred-thousand-hour life span, your new LED holiday lights could last until the next century.

Ribbons and Bows

Instead of tying ribbons on your holiday packages this year, garnish them with recyclable paper bows (natural-fiber raffia), dried flowers, or a reusable scarf. If two out of three households conserved an arm's length of ribbon, the amount saved could tie a bow around the earth.

Wrapping Paper

Cut back on wrapping waste by placing gifts in reusable bags or baskets. If you prefer traditional wrapping paper, try to find a brand with recycled content and then reuse any large pieces to wrap presents again next year. Between Thanksgiving and New Year's, Americans produce an extra two billion pounds of garbage per week, much of which is gift packaging. If 40 percent of U.S. households reduced their holiday paper consumption by just two sheets this year, the savings could gift-wrap Manhattan Island.

Wine and Beer

Beverage Packaging

The energy required to produce a single twelve-ounce aluminum can from virgin ore is enough to produce nearly two new twelve-ounce glass bottles. So the next time you buy a six-pack of beer, opt for glass bottles over aluminum cans. The manufacturing energy conserved could power your television through two Sunday NFL games. If 10 percent of beer drinkers replaced a six-pack of cans with six glass bottles, the energy saved could fly thirty thousand Cowboys fans from Dallas to the Meadowlands to watch their team take on the New York Giants.

Domestic vs. Imported

If you have the option, buy from a nearby winery or microbrewery. Your purchase will reduce fossil fuel consumption because you're buying local and yield the additional benefit of supporting your local community. There are an estimated 176 million adult beer and wine drinkers in the United States, who collectively consume about 6.5 billion gallons of beer and 690 million gallons of wine per year.

Organic Wine

Organic wines can be affordable, tasty, and healthy alternatives to their nonorganic counterparts. A bottle of conventionally produced wine may contain up to 250 different types of chemicals. If you're a wine connoisseur, a year's worth of organic wine purchases would keep roughly 2 pounds of fertilizers and 50 grams of pesticides out of the environment (and out of your wineglass). If one in twenty wine drinkers decided to demand organic wines only, organic vineyards would increase by nearly forty thousand acres, resulting in the elimination of more than 3.3 million pounds of agrochemicals per year.

Motor Vehicles

Biodiesel

If your vehicle has a diesel engine, consider using biodiesel. Not only is biodiesel more energy efficient than other fuels, it's renewable, biodegradable, and free of the sulfur pollutants characteristic of traditional petrodiesel. If you were to begin using biodiesel B20 (a fuel containing 20 percent biodiesel) instead of conventional diesel, you would conserve an average of 50 gallons of petroleum per year and reduce your carbon emissions by 30 percent. If all diesel cars sold this year used B20 fuel, the annual savings would equal 23.8 million gallons of petrodiesel—enough to transport more than nine hundred thousand children to school and back for an entire year.

Fuel

Don't bother buying the more expensive high-octane fuel unless your owner's manual specifically recommends it. If your vehicle was made to run on 87 octane and you choose 92 octane, there will be no improvement to your engine power, fuel efficiency, speed, or performance. The price difference per fill-up, however, amounts to an extra gallon of gasoline. If all drivers used lower-grade octane, $3 billion per year would be saved—enough to buy more than 107,000 hybrid cars.

Hybrid

If you're planning to buy a new car, consider buying a hybrid. You could conserve more than twenty gallons (an entire tank) of gasoline per month than the average vehicle. If an additional 1 percent of vehicles sold in the United States per year were hybrids, the gasoline saved annually would fill nearly 4,600 tanker trucks.

Oil

Ask for rerefined motor oil the next time you change the oil in your car. The production of five quarts of high-quality rerefined lubricating oil uses only two gallons of used oil, whereas producing and refining five quarts of virgin oil requires two barrels of crude oil. If 5 percent of households began using rerefined oil for oil changes, 2.5 billion gallons of oil could be conserved per year.

PZEV

Partial zero-emission vehicles (PZEVs) run at least 90 percent cleaner than the average new car. If you buy a PZEV, you'll release only about one pound of smog-causing emissions per fifteen thousand miles driven. If all new motor vehicles sold within the Los Angeles basin over the next fifteen years were PZEV, the smog problem would disappear.

Services

The next time you need a rental car, taxi, or limo service, try to choose a hybrid or other low-emission vehicle. A fifty-mile trip in a hybrid vehicle will use less than one gallon of gasoline, whereas the same trip in a standard sedan may consume more than twice that amount. If 20 percent of U.S. car rental transactions were for hybrids, a total of fifty million gallons of gasoline annually would be saved. This much fuel is nearly enough to run the entire fleet of New York City taxis for a full year.

Tires

When it's time for you to buy new tires, consider retreads. Retread tires are equal in safety and performance to new tires but use only one-third of the petroleum resources to produce and cost roughly $48 less per tire. If you buy four retread tires instead of four new ones, you'll help conserve 60 gallons of oil and could save nearly $200 in tire costs. If demand for retread tires were to increase by 10 percent, the total oil savings per year would be about 290 million gallons, which is more gasoline than all the cars in the United States use per day, about $900 million worth.

Used Vehicles

If you buy a used vehicle instead of a new one, you'll help save energy as well as over 2,150 pounds of steel. Nine percent of the energy used by a car over its lifetime is consumed in the manufacturing process. If one in a hundred potential new-car buyers chose to purchase a used car instead, the amount of steel saved annually could reconstruct the Golden Gate Bridge—twice a year.

Luxury Items

Boats

If you're planning to buy a boat, the best ones for the environment have oars and sails. Electric motors are the next best choice. If you buy a diesel-powered vessel, however, choose a four-stroke engine or a two-stroke engine with direct fuel injection (DFI). These engines will use 35 to 50 percent less gasoline than conventional two-stroke engines, which are inefficient and discharge up to one-third of the fuel in your tank (unburned) into the water. If every boat with a two-stroke engine were eventually replaced with a four-stroke or DFI, the reduction in the quantity of raw fuel emitted into the America's lakes and rivers would be equivalent to preventing fifteen *Exxon Valdez* oil spills every year.

China

If you prefer fine bone china (made from 50 percent animal bone ash) or porcelain china, select a variety that's dishwasher safe. You'll save roughly 35 gallons of water by washing eight five-piece place settings in a dishwasher instead of by hand. If an additional 1 percent of engaged couples registered for dishwasher-safe china, a total of 1.75 million gallons of water would be saved after every dinner party.

Crystal

If you buy crystal, choose lead-free varieties. The lead content of a beverage stored in a standard crystal decanter can be 130 times higher than the EPA standard for lead in drinking water. Not only is lead exposure highly toxic to humans, but the environmental effects of lead mining can last for millennia. Groundwater supplies in Wales, famous for its crystal making, continue to be polluted by lead mines excavated more than two thousand years ago.

Diamonds

Buy a vintage diamond instead of a new one. You'll save all the energy and mining costs associated with bringing a new stone to market. This adds up to a savings of 171 gallons of water, thirty-five kilowatt-hours of electricity, and 1 gallon of petroleum—per carat.

Gold Jewelry

Consider buying antique, recycled, or vintage jewelry. The mining required to produce a typical .33-ounce eighteen-karat-gold band uses more than 13,000 gallons of water and leaves twenty tons of cyanide-laden mine sludge. If just one in one thousand households opted for antique, recycled, or vintage jewelry for its next purchase, the savings would total two million tons of mine waste—roughly the total weight of 26.7 million American adults—and 1.37 billion gallons of water.

Motorcycles

If the option is available to you, look for an electric or hybrid motorcycle. Standard two-stroke motorcycles emit up to twenty-five times more pollution per mile than passenger cars. Your next best choice is a four-stroke engine, which will improve your fuel economy by 25 percent and halve your emissions over the two-stroke model. On average, if you buy a four-stroke motorcycle, you'll save about nine gallons of gas per year—enough to take one more road trip from Phoenix to Las Vegas and back. If 15 percent of motorcycle owners chose four-stroke engines for their next purchase, the energy saved could light the Las Vegas strip for an entire year.

Motor Homes

If you've got your eye fixed on a plush twenty-nine-foot motor home and are planning to travel in it for most of the year, you can save money on the purchase price, maintenance, and fuel costs by choosing an equivalently luxurious twenty-six-foot sport utility recreational vehicle to tow behind a truck. Not only can you get twice the gas mileage by towing, but you'll be able to detach the trailer and use the truck for short trips. On average, a motor home will get seven to eight miles per gallon, while a truck towing a fifth wheel or trailer can achieve fourteen to fifteen miles per gallon. Over the course of a year and eight thousand miles driven, this comes to a total savings of more than five hundred gallons of fuel and up to $1,500.

Silver

If you choose a sturdy set of flatware made from stainless steel instead of sterling silver, you'll not only save significant cash, but you'll save the energy of mining silver ore. Since most stainless steel is made from recycled materials, eight five-piece place settings of stainless flatware will save more than 1,300 kilowatt-hours of energy. The value of this energy could buy a nice $100 stainless fondue set to match. If just .5 percent of newlyweds chose stainless flatware over sterling, the energy saved could entertain twenty-two million fondue parties.

Electronics

Computers

Look for Energy Star–qualified computers, which adjust to a low power mode when not in use. This feature reduces the computer's energy consumption by up to 70 percent and can also make the equipment run cooler and last longer. If one-quarter of U.S. households eventually replaced conventional computers with those that are Energy Star qualified, the energy saved over the computers' lifetimes could light every U.S. household for more than a year.

DVD Players

If your next DVD player is Energy Star qualified, you'll save roughly 30 kilowatt-hours of energy per year over a conventional unit. If every DVD player sold this year were Energy Star rated, the annual energy saved would equal 837 million kilowatt-hours—equivalent to the amount generated by a nuclear power plant over a forty-day period.

Fax Machines

If you haven't gone completely paperless with the use of Internet faxing, you can conserve office space, power, and manufacturing waste by choosing a fax machine that also serves as a printer, copier, and scanner.

By purchasing a single all-in-one model instead of three or four separate devices, you'll save about 400 kilowatt-hours of electricity per year. If one in one hundred households with home offices were to use all-in-one fax machines instead of individual fax, copy, and printing units, 136 million kilowatt-hours of total energy could be saved per year—enough to fax nearly all of the 7.5 billion pages of archived, original office documents generated annually around the world.

Laptops vs. Desktops

If you're planning to buy a new computer, consider getting a laptop or notebook instead of a desktop. Laptops require fewer materials and less energy to produce than desktops and use a fraction of the electricity to run. If you choose a laptop over a desktop, you'll save an average of 220 kilowatt-hours per year and about $20 on your annual electricity bill. If one in twenty-three households made its next computer purchase a laptop instead of a desktop, the energy saved could keep the lights on for every household in Silicon Valley.

Mobile Phones

Try to limit the frequency with which you replace your cell phone, and make sure you e-cycle (dispose of it through an electronic waste management company) or donate your old one. If you keep each mobile phone you buy for three years instead of just eighteen months, you'll effectively cut the resources needed to make a new one. If just 10 percent of cell phone users kept their next phone for three years before replacing it, an average of 5.2 million phones could be saved from disposal each year.

Personal Digital Assistants

You can save energy if you avoid buying PDAs with features that you don't need, especially if you have other devices to serve those purposes (playing music, viewing digital pictures, text messaging, and so on). You can send and receive more than seventeen e-mails on your BlackBerry™ for the amount of energy required to send and receive one e-mail on a color-screen PDA. Or with the energy consumed to play two minutes of music on a PDA, you could play twelve minutes of music on a simple MP3 player. PDAs use three times more power than a cell phone to send a text message. Lower power requirements mean longer battery life and less money spent over the life of the product.

Phones

If you need to buy a new phone for a bedroom or home office, consider buying one with a cord. You'll save about 28 kilowatt-hours of energy per phone annually. Standard corded phones consume little energy, while cordless units draw constant power during charging and standby modes. If 5 percent of U.S. households chose one corded phone over a cordless model, the energy savings would total 140 million kilowatt-hours annually—enough talk time to keep 130,000 teens' phone lines busy for every waking hour of the summer.

Refurbished Computers

Think about buying a refurbished computer. You'll save the 139 pounds of waste, 7,300 gallons of water, and 2,300 kilowatt-hours of energy associated with manufacturing a new one. If just 1 percent of the twenty million computers that become obsolete each year were replaced with refurbished machines, the waste saved could fill more than 1,700 garbage trucks; the water conserved could fill seventy-three thousand backyard swimming pools; and the energy saved could power every personal computer owned in the United States for fifty-five straight hours.

Stereos

Instead of buying a traditional home stereo that plays tapes and compact discs—both of which are quickly becoming obsolete—choose audio equipment that's compatible with your MP3 player. These digital systems are not only less expensive than the all-in-one units, but they're smaller, which means less waste overall.

Televisions

If you're planning to upgrade your television to a flat screen, you can save roughly 275 kilowatt-hours of energy and $25 per year by choosing a thirty-two-inch LCD panel over an equal-size plasma screen. If five in one hundred households made this choice, the total energy saved could power each of the 266 million televisions owned in the United States through forty straight hours of the next *Twilight Zone* marathon.

Video Game Consoles

If you're thinking of purchasing a video game system, consider buying a preowned one. You'll prevent nine pounds of plastics and hazardous materials from potentially entering a landfill as well as save the resources and energy used to manufacture and transport a new one. If just one in fifty new video game consoles purchased per year were preowned, it would save 2.28 million pounds of electronic waste per year from entering landfills.

"My approach to living green is all about keeping it simple. Be mindful of the impact your actions leave behind, take responsibility for your actions, and have respect for the world around you.

I'm into saving, and I've always been thrifty. The beautiful thing is conserving and saving money go hand in hand. My green tips would be to take short showers, turn off the faucet when you brush your teeth, use a water filter instead of drinking bottled water, and flush only when necessary. Turning out the lights whenever you leave a room makes a small difference, too. All of these little things make a big difference. Details matter and the girls in the Top Model house will tell you nothing makes me crazier than wasting resources. It's not that they have to do everything I do, but if I can set an example of how to look and feel, I can also help set an example about how to be friendlier to the planet. Everyone can. And if we all practice these habits, we can make the planet look gooood!

I'm not saying you have to be a hippie, but if you want to, let your freak-flag fly! What's key is to care about yourself, care about your family, care about your friends, and care about the world. Everything comes full circle."

8

health and beauty

Mirror, Mirror, on the Wall,
Who's the Greenest of Them All?

THE BIG PICTURE

Looking good can turn out to be very bad for you—and the planet.

The health and beauty industry is a $160 billion-a-year business and isn't particularly concerned about slim packaging or losing pounds when it comes to toxins in their products. Even natural skin care products need only 1 percent natural ingredients in order to be called "natural"; the rest can be man-made. Since you absorb up to 60 percent of any substance applied to your skin, you could absorb up to 4.4 pounds of man-made chemicals through your body every year.

Not pretty. And although not everyone walks around with more plaster on their face than a mannequin, we do spend lots of time and money trying to look good. Americans spend seven times more money per year on beauty products than the federal government spends on education.

A lot of the cost for us (and for the environment) is packaging, big packaging. How much perfume is really inside that big bottle inside that even bigger box that you put inside your shopping bag? Big packaging is mostly a marketing tool. Consider this: Each of us consumes about two hundred pounds of plastic per year, and about sixty pounds of it is packaging that we just throw away.

Of course, it isn't just beauty products we're talking about here; it's the everyday hygienic stuff that we can get lost in. More than two billion disposable razors are purchased every year. And they aren't purchased to be held on to (they're labeled "disposable" for a reason). That means all those plastic handles and metal blades end up in the trash. They most likely sit next to the more than fifty million pounds of used toothbrushes that end up in landfills each year, too. Most shampoo bottles are made from virgin plastic. Conditioners and body washes aren't any better for the planet. Soaps are even being scoured for some of their more harmful additives. And then there's deodorant/antiperspirant, which is made from the astringent salts of aluminum, zinc, or zirconium to seal up pores and reduce sweat output. The type of mined aluminum used scars the landscape, pollutes water, and consumes vast amounts of electricity.

But listen, we aren't saying don't brush, don't shave, and be stinky—especially after a workout at the gym—just be mindful.

And speaking of the gym, there are about forty million or so people who belong to a gym in the United States. They use water, towels, water bottles, and little plastic drink cups in repetition. Ironically, however, it takes four ounces of water in the manufacturing process to make a three-ounce drink cup. That ought to make you think twice the next time you take one from the bubbler and toss it right away. And in just one day, the gym towels used are enough to wrap around Arnold Schwarzenegger's chest at the height of his bodybuilding career 37.5 million times.

Keeping all that in mind, we've created the "Simple Steps" to be just that. Taking into account all the points of the Big Picture, they give you the biggest impact with the least amount of effort.

The Simple Steps

1. Bring your own reusable water bottle filled with filtered water from home every time you go to the gym. You could save an average of $200 per year as well as 14 pounds of plastic. If one in twenty gym members who generally buy a bottle of water before each workout brought a reusable water bottle from home, the plastic saved annually would total nearly 29 million pounds, a weight that would take two hundred thousand people each bench-pressing 150 pounds to lift.

2. Buy a quality razor with refillable blades. Disposable plastic razors are neither recyclable nor biodegradable, and they take significantly more energy to produce. If for the next year you replaced your purchases of disposable razors with refill cartridges, the amount of energy saved by not manufacturing the extra plastic could brew you five pots of coffee. If half of the disposable razors sold per year were replaced with refills, the energy saved could fly twenty-six thousand San Diego java lovers to pick their own Kona coffee on the Big Island of Hawaii.

3. If the weather's right, consider giving the treadmill a rest and taking your walking or jogging routine outdoors. A 25 percent shift in time on the treadmill to time outside would conserve about sixty kilowatt-hours of energy per year. If an additional 10 percent of Americans who walk as their number one form of physical activity walked outside instead of indoors, it would save as much energy as it would take to drive a car forty thousand miles. Put another way, that's the total distance the contestants on *The Amazing Race* travel around the world throughout the series.

THE LITTLE THINGS

At the Gym

Equipment

Try to do your cardio workouts on equipment that doesn't require an external power supply. Choose, for example, a stationary bike or elliptical machine over a treadmill or stair-climber. For a forty-minute workout, you could save 0.8 kilowatt-hour of energy—the amount you'd burn if you ran seven miles. If for a whole year you stayed off the treadmill and rode the bike five times per week instead, you'd save 160 kilowatt-hours of energy—roughly what you'd expend by running the length of Interstate 5 from Mexico to the Canadian border.

Sauna/Steamroom

Try to shut off the sauna when you're through using it. Even if a timer is set to shut it off automatically, you'll conserve about 0.1 kilowatt of energy for every minute the sauna is not running. If half of the saunas in the United States were turned off for just one additional minute per day, the annual savings would total close to 70 million kilowatt-hours of energy per year. This is enough to cool nearly twenty-five thousand homes for an entire hot, humid East Coast summer.

Showering

If you routinely shower before work in the morning and then again after your evening visit to the gym, consider switching to a morning workout and showering just once a day. You'll save about two hundred gallons of water for each shower you subtract from your schedule. Over the course of a year, you could save more than thirty thousand gallons of water—enough to fill a twenty-by-forty-foot backyard swimming pool.

Towels

Bring your own workout towel instead of using one that your gym provides. You'll not only reduce your exposure to harsh detergents, bleaches, and other disinfectants, but you'll help save water and energy as well. If just 1 percent of fitness club members in the United States were to start bringing their own workout towels, four thousand fewer loads of laundry would have to be washed per day—an annual savings of more than thirty-six million gallons of water.

Outdoor Exercise

Biking

Bike in the morning and stay on marked paths. You can minimize your intake of fumes by staying on the edge of traffic zones, such as in bike lanes or on bike paths, and you can reduce your exposure to air pollutants by doing the majority of your outdoor exercise in the morning, when pollution levels are lowest.

Hiking

Minimize the impact of hiking activities by leaving behind only footprints and keeping those footprints on established trails. In the United States each year, over two hundred thousand miles of trails are trodden by some seventy-five million American hikers. Collectively, they could make a boot print twice the size of the president's 125-acre Camp David compound.

Swimming

If you have a choice, swim in a saltwater (saline) or solar-ionized pool instead of a chlorinated one. Swimming pools that are sterilized with salts or ionization are not only better for the environment, they're better for your skin, eyes, hair, and lungs. If all chlorinated swimming pools in the

United States were to convert to saline, it would eliminate 182 million pounds of pool chemicals per year.

In Front of the Mirror and in the Bathroom

Baby Oil

Try choosing oils made from the seeds of fruits and nuts instead of from the refinement of petroleum. Baby oil, or mineral oil, is a by-product of gasoline production. About one hundred million gallons of mineral oil are used each year in the United States—an amount equal to about 25 percent of the U.S. daily consumption of gas.

Bath Salts/Bubble Bath

If you buy bath salts or bubble bath, try to buy concentrated varieties. For example, bubble bath brands that recommend one tablespoon (one-half ounce, or one capful) per bath will last twice as long as those that suggest one ounce (two capfuls) per bath. If you buy a sixteen-ounce plastic bottle of bubble bath every other month and switched to a more concentrated version, you could save about one-quarter pound of plastic and $10 to $20 per year or more. If one in one hundred households decreased its bubble bath purchases in this way, the savings would total 250,000 pounds of plastic. This much plastic could build a wading pool the size of Wrigley Field.

Conditioner

Consider using a two-in-one shampoo and conditioner instead of buying each separately. You'll not only save on money and packaging, but you'll likely save additional time, water, and money by reducing the length of your shower. If one in seven U.S. households replaced its shampoo and conditioner purchase with a single two-in-one bottle, the amount of plastic saved per year could fill a football field twenty-seven stories high.

Cotton Balls

Check to make sure the cotton balls you buy are actually made from cotton, as some cotton balls contain polyester. The production of polyester—a synthetic material that's related to plastic—uses 67 percent more energy than the production of cotton. Also, consider looking for organic cotton balls or cotton balls bleached without chlorine, which are better for the health of your family as well as for the environment.

Deodorant

When you buy deodorant, try to avoid antiperspirants, which use aluminum salts to seal up your pores. In addition to being a potential health toxin, aluminum takes a tremendous amount of energy to mine. If you buy one stick of aluminum-free deodorant, the energy saved could power your laptop for thirty minutes. If 5 percent of adults switched from antiperspirants for good, the value of the annual energy savings could buy 250 new computers for U.S. classrooms every year.

Eyeliner

You can minimize waste by buying eyeliner pencils encased in wood instead of pencils or liquids contained within plastic. Wood shavings have the potential to biodegrade, whereas most plastics do not. If one in twenty eyeliner users switched from using plastic-encased pencils to wooden ones, nearly ten thousand pounds of plastic could be saved.

Eye Shadow

If you use pressed eye shadow, choose a brand that provides a reusable compact with slots for refills. Each time you buy a refill instead of an entirely new container, you'll reduce your costs, the amount of energy used to produce and ship the hard plastic, glass, or chrome packaging (some of which come with mirrors), and the amount of waste you discard when it's empty. If one in twenty-five women chose refillable eye shadow, more than 350,000 pounds of wasted cosmetics containers could be saved each year.

Foundation

Opt for foundation in a simple recyclable (or reusable) glass container over one sold in a nonrecyclable plastic tube or bottle. The manufacturing energy saved by avoiding the plastic container could run the light bulb in your makeup mirror for more than seven hours. If one in twenty women chose glass over plastic packaging for her next foundation purchase, the energy conserved could fill a twenty-gallon gas tank once a week for twenty-four years.

Hair Dye

If you purchase at-home hair color, you may be gentler on the environment by choosing semi- or demi-permanent dyes with plant-based pigments as opposed to permanent varieties with synthetic dyes.

Lipstick

Given that the average woman may inadvertently ingest more than four pounds of lipstick in her lifetime, you'll want to look for lip color made from plant-derived ingredients instead of from synthetic oils, paraffin waxes, and toxic coal tar dyes (look for FD&C or D&C followed by a color and number). If one in five lipstick wearers began demanding plant-based options, total petroleum product consumption would decrease by more than 825,000 pounds per year.

Lotions

If the lotion you usually buy comes with a pump dispenser, you can avoid sending another hand pump to the landfill by purchasing a refill container with a flip top and just reusing your empty bottle. If 10 percent of U.S. households made a onetime purchase of a lotion bottle without an attached pump, the plastic saved would be an estimated 250,000 pounds—enough lotion pumps to fill nearly 1,200 tanning booths from floor to ceiling.

Mascara

Your best choice for mascara is one that is made from plants and minerals instead of from petroleum products. However, if this is not a viable option for you, avoid varieties that come in plastic bubble packs on cardboard backings. This unnecessary waste contributes to the fact that more than a quarter of the volume of America's trash is packaging—525 pounds per person per year on average.

Perfume/Cologne

Try switching to a perfume or cologne that contains natural, pure botanical ingredients. Most conventional fragranced products contain chemicals derived from petroleum and are linked negatively to environmental health effects. Because eight hundred million pounds of these chemicals are used per year to make fragranced products, they are considered to be one of the most prevalent toxins in the environment.

Shampoo

Look for shampoo bottles made from postconsumer recycled plastic, which helps reuse plastic and cuts down on waste. Also, it takes less energy to make recycled plastic than it does to make virgin plastic. For example, if you buy a single thirteen-ounce shampoo bottle that contains 25 percent postconsumer materials, the energy saved would be enough to blow-dry your hair for ten minutes. If one in ten U.S. households purchased shampoo in a bottle made from recycled materials, the energy conserved could wind-power 160 homes for an entire year.

Shaving Gel/Foam

If you choose to buy shaving gel (as opposed to just using soap or body wash), avoid the aerosol variety. Although aerosol chemicals no longer deplete the ozone layer, those chemicals have been replaced by petroleum propellants that are discharged with the foamy product you rub onto your skin. If your household refuses to buy aerosol shaving products, you could reduce your direct consumption of petroleum by nearly one-half pound per year. If 10 percent of households chose alternatives to aerosol shave gels and foams, the petroleum savings from the propellants alone could light 270,000 households for a month.

Soap

Use bars of soap versus liquid wash. It's less expensive, and it saves packaging waste. The average bar of soap lasts for about twenty showers, whereas a sixteen-ounce bottle of body wash lasts for an average of eighty showers. But body wash costs on average more than four times as much as soap. If every U.S. household replaced a bottle of body wash with a bar of soap, roughly 2.5 million pounds of plastic containers could be diverted from the waste stream.

Sponges

Instead of buying a synthetic nylon sponge, consider using a completely natural and biodegradable loofah or a plain reusable washcloth. Since nylon is made from petroleum and can't be recycled, you'll conserve the energy used to make it, as well as the environmental cost of disposing of it. If one in fifty Americans used a sustainable alternative to the nylon puff, it would save a sponge big enough to sop up almost a million-square-foot flood of water.

Tampons

Try to buy organic tampons. The pesticides and bleaches used in conventional cotton tampons are pollutants in air, water, and soil. If just one in twenty women switched to organic tampons, we could eliminate 750,000 pounds of pesticides annually.

"Most people know my major sponsor on the NASCAR circuit is Budweiser. They've been with me since 1999, and we've won a lot of races like the Daytona 500 together.

What a lot of people don't know—and I didn't, either, until recently—are some of the things Anheuser-Busch (the company that has produced Budweiser for more than 125 years) does to help the world. Anheuser-Busch is one of the largest recyclers of aluminum cans on the planet. They actually recycle more cans than they sell. And they have reduced the amount of aluminum in each can to save more natural resources. They also get involved in protecting wildlife habitat with the 'Bud Outdoors' program.

These are things they don't advertise. They do it because it's the right thing to do, which I respect. So recycle your Budweiser cans the next time you and your buddies get together for some cold ones. Chances are, within about sixty days, the cans you recycled will hit the shelves again so you can enjoy a few more Buds the next time my red No. 8 car and I cross the finish line first."

sports

Take Me Out to the Ball Game, but First Let Me Grab My Water Bottle

THE BIG PICTURE

More than 350 million pairs of athletic shoes are sold in the United States every year. These 700 million new soles tread around four hundred miles before they wear out. Then they are laid to rest in the trash.

The environmental footprint of sports goes beyond shoes, however. Bats, helmets, balls, gloves, shin pads, and other types of sports equipment are often made from PVC, a widely used type of plastic that can be hard or soft but can't be easily recycled. Not that much sports equipment is ever really in a position to be recycled; most of it lies around in garages, closets, and attics and is rarely used.

Sure, you can use your old tennis balls to play with man's best friend, but the thirty million new balls made every year are mostly packed in pressured plastic tubes, which don't make for such great fetch toys. And that means they end up in the can along with the sixty million plastic water bottles we throw away each day.

As most athletes will tell you, water is a must in the sports world— it replenishes the body. The land on which sports are played needs replenishment, too, however, and that requires a lot more H_2O. The world's golf courses use 2.5 billion gallons of water a day for irrigation. This same amount of water is also needed to support 4.7 billion people per day—pretty close to the entire world's population. Golf courses also use pesticides and fertilizers that contribute to water pollution.

But let's not take swings at just the golf community. Skiers, hockey players, and swimmers also play in, on, and with the world's water supply. And field sports trounce the land—not just during the day, but at night, too. Night games also cause light pollution. In fact, overillumination is responsible for approximately two million barrels of oil per day in wasted energy.

Keeping all that in mind, we've created the "Simple Steps" to be just that. Taking into account all the points of the Big Picture, they give you the biggest impact with the least amount of effort.

The Simple Steps

1. **Consider renting or leasing sports equipment on a per use basis** as opposed to wasting money and cluttering up your garage with gear that you know you won't be able to enjoy more than once or twice a year. You'll reduce the energy needed to produce an additional piece of equipment and decrease the amount of waste eventually sent to the landfill. If one-eighth of the skis and snowboards that are purchased each year were rented instead, they could be lined up from the Riviera on the Mediterranean Sea to Slovenia on the Balkan peninsula and trace the entire five-hundred-mile crescent of the Alps.

2. **Try to buy athletic shoes and hiking boots made with recycled rubber soles** in order to help reduce waste and save energy. (Ask your retailer about specific brands that do this.) The energy saved by producing a single pair of athletic soles made from 25 percent recy-

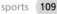

cled rubber could power your television through more than eleven hours of Indiana Pacers basketball. If every athletic shoe sold this year had a sole containing 25 percent recycled rubber, the rubber savings could produce an additional ninety-two million pairs of rubber soles. If shipped to Indianapolis, they could fill the entire volume of Conseco Fieldhouse.

3. When you play outdoor sports, try not to litter and go the extra mile by picking up and properly disposing of any trash you see. If every sports fan picked up and properly disposed of just one piece of litter per year, more than 1,480 tons, or enough to fill 185 garbage trucks, of unsightly trash could be removed from trails, beaches, lakes, rivers, forests, oceans, and other fragile ecosystems.

THE LITTLE THINGS

Equipment

Bags

Choose duffel bags and backpacks made from recycled materials over those made from petroleum-derived virgin polyester or PVC, which is less recyclable. For each bag purchased, you could save the equivalent of fifteen two-liter soda bottles from entering landfills. If 1 percent of Americans who participate in outdoor activities each year were to purchase a sports bag made from recycled materials, more than 180,000 pounds of plastic could be diverted from the trash.

Balls

If you buy tennis balls (for yourself or your dog), consider purchasing the pressureless variety. Pressureless tennis balls are not only longer lasting than their pressurized counterparts, but are sold in a recyclable paper box or a reusable mesh bag instead of the pressurized plastic or metal tube with the aluminum seal. If you generally buy a dozen balls per month, you can save more than three pounds of plastic a year. If an additional 25 percent of the 360 million tennis balls manufactured each year were pressureless, the plastic tubes saved could form a line from Queens, New York, to Wimbledon.

Bats

Since aluminum is the most energy intensive of all materials manufactured in the United States, consider using a bat made of renewable wood or even bamboo. You'll help reduce pollution and conserve the energy equivalent of almost a gallon of gasoline per bat (based on how much energy it takes to make one). If one in ten Little League players opted for nonaluminum bats, the total energy saved could transport ten thousand fans from all over the country to watch the Little League World Series Championship game in South Williamsport, Pennsylvania.

Bicycles

Choose a bike with a steel frame over an aluminum frame and you'll conserve at least twenty-five kilowatt-hours of energy. Steel frames can be made with recycled materials, whereas aluminum frames must be manufactured from new, virgin ore and therefore require more energy to make. Steel frames that are not made from recycled steel, however, still conserve energy over those made from aluminum. If an additional 10 percent of bicycles sold per year carried steel frames instead of aluminum ones, four million pedals would be put to the metal, saving the energy equivalent of a year's worth of gas for 2,400 cars.

Donate

Donate your used sporting goods. You'll not only contribute to a good cause, save resources in the manufacturing of new equipment, and delay the landfilling of your old gear, but you'll get a tax write-off as well. If 10 percent of American golfers donated a set of fourteen clubs to the Goodwill, the total tax rebate could fill each of the more than 270,000 golf holes in courses around the country with more than one hundred golf balls (which would require digging some deeper holes!).

Equipment—General

Look for lighter-weight items, such as bats, rackets, bikes, sticks, or clubs, which are made from composite resins. They are more durable than their wood or metal counterparts and help conserve resources, save production energy, and reduce the amount of waste sent to landfills.

Equipment—Used

Try purchasing used equipment. The market for used equipment is already near $1 billion and represents the resale of hundreds of thousands of skis, golf clubs, treadmills, camping gear, and exercise bikes. If 5 percent of the money spent on new sporting goods were directed at used goods instead, Americans could save $250 million per year, enough to buy solar panels for twenty thousand houses.

Gloves and Mitts

Avoid any gloves or mitts made from vinyl or PVC plastic. PVC production can contribute to both air and water pollution. Plus, PVC is energy intensive to recycle and is highly toxic when burned. The production of 168,000 pounds of PVC (and the associated environmental effects) could be prevented if 10 percent of Little League players' first gloves were made from nonvinyl materials.

Golf Clubs

Unfortunately, golf loses about as many players as it attracts each year. So if you're a golf novice and are planning to buy new clubs, start off with just a half set of irons. As you improve your swing, you can add to your set. But if you decide golf isn't your game, you'll have spent only a fraction of the cost and used a fraction of the resources in the end. If 50 percent of new golfers bought only a half set of clubs, the materials saved could rebuild the Seattle Space Needle every year.

Helmets

Look for helmets made from materials that can eventually be reused or recycled and you'll help reduce the volume of nonbiodegradable landfill waste. If one in twenty U.S. children who ride bicycles used helmets made from recyclable materials, 175,000 pounds of bicycle helmets could be saved from landfills every year. If this material were formed into one giant helmet, it would cover the entire half-mile racetrack and infield of the Bristol Motor Speedway.

Surfboards

Help reduce waste by purchasing surfboards made from recyclable materials (such as polystyrene foam) and covered with an epoxy resin, rather than those made from other materials and covered with polyester and fiberglass. Epoxy boards are not only lighter, but tend to last five times longer. If just one in fifty surfers in the world ensured that their next board purchased was made from recyclable polystyrene, the number of surfboards saved from landfills could stretch more than 2,400 miles, from Waimea Bay, Hawaii, to Ocean Beach, California.

Tennis Rackets

Instead of choosing a racket strung with nonrenewable fibers such as nylon or polyester, select one with natural strings. If an additional 20 percent of all new tennis rackets sold per year contained natural strings instead of synthetic ones, which are usually made from petroleum, it could save the energy equivalent of over 22,500 gallons of gasoline and reduce annually the use of twenty-five thousand pounds of synthetic material. This represents the strings of eight hundred thousand rackets.

Water Bottles

Refill your water bottle. If just two out of three sports fans refilled a water bottle rather than buying a new one, it would save about as many plastic bottles as there are people in the United States.

Yoga Mats

Buy yoga mats made from plant-based materials such as natural rubber, jute, or cotton instead of petroleum-derived plastics or other synthetics. Avoid especially any yoga mats containing environmentally toxic PVC. If every yoga enthusiast in the United States purchased a natural yoga mat instead of one made from PVC plastic, collectively they could prevent the production and eventual landfilling of 46.2 million pounds of PVC plastic. If these mats were laid flat and stacked, they would reach more than seven times the height of Mount Everest.

Playing and Participating

Baseball/Softball

You can save energy by scheduling daytime games for your baseball and softball leagues. A single field can use an average of seventy-two thousand kilowatt-hours of energy annually for nighttime lighting. This much energy could keep your house lit for sixty years. In the United States, there are more than thirty-three million youth and adults who belong to organized baseball and softball teams. If just 10 percent of these teams rescheduled one evening game for a daylight hour, the energy saved could broadcast the Major League Baseball All-Star Game on eleven million televisions.

Basketball

Take your daytime pickup game outside. You'll save energy as well as wear and tear on the indoor court. Gymnasium lighting can consume over sixty thousand kilowatt-hours of energy per year, much of which is used unnecessarily during the day. Or if you get the chance, check out one of the more than one hundred basketball courts around the country made from the soles of recycled athletic shoes. They're cropping up in most major cities, including Chicago, Washington, D.C., Atlanta, Miami, San Francisco, and Los Angeles. The total number of shoes that have gone into these courts is three times the number that participate in the New York City Marathon each year.

Cycling

Try to recycle your old bicycle tires and inner tubes instead of throwing them away. You'll prevent about two pounds of rubber from being landfilled and may help provide materials for a new handbag, a pair of hiking boots, or even a bike path itself. If one in fourteen American cyclists were to recycle his or her bicycle tires each year, the rubber saved could pave the current route of the Tour de France.

Football and Soccer

If you have the choice between playing on grass or artificial turf, choose grass. Natural grass is renewable, and clippings can be composted. Grasses produce oxygen, remove air pollutants, filter rainwater, facilitate groundwater recharge, and maintain cool surface temperatures. Artificial turf production is energy intensive and uses synthetic materials, some of which are recycled but none of which are recyclable. While some artificial fields may require less maintenance than natural fields, they last only for an average of ten years before they need to be pulled up and taken to the landfill.

Golf

Try visiting some of the hundreds of conservation-minded golf courses in the United States that have committed to decreasing water consumption, reducing chemicals, preserving native landscapes, and protecting wildlife habitats. Irrigation improvements alone can save a course an average of 1.9 million gallons of water per year. If an additional 1 percent of the sixteen thousand golf courses in the United States adopted water conservation strategies, the annual water savings could restore a wetland the size of Augusta National Golf Club.

Hockey

Try to schedule your ice times in the evenings, when energy costs are lowest. If you're renting the rink after hours, see if the facility will allow the ice temperature to rise one degree. The ice will still be frozen, but you'll impose less of a burden on the refrigeration system and conserve energy. In fact, merely allowing ice temperatures to rise by one degree at night can save an ice rink around twenty-one thousand kilowatt-hours of energy per year—as much as your refrigerator will consume over its entire lifetime. If every ice rink in the United States and Canada employed this energy conservation measure, the money saved could buy nearly four thousand NHL season ticket packages for behind-the-glass seats.

Skiing/Snowboarding

When skiing or snowboarding, make sure you stay on established slopes and trails and avoid venturing onto ecologically sensitive terrain. You'll help preserve the remaining natural landscapes and native habitats and reduce the rate of erosion in these areas. And if all 12.9 million skiers and snowboarders followed these guidelines, they'd likely prevent many of the more than thirty thousand injuries that occur each winter from these sports.

Surfing

When you're vying for better beach access, always keep your vehicle on paved roads or marked pathways, and never drive across sand dunes. You'll save on gasoline, protect coastal habitats, prevent coastal erosion, and ensure a future of good surf. If you and the other estimated four million surfers in the United States stood shoulder to shoulder, there would be enough of you to trace the entire 1,340-mile California coastline. So it's important to vary your surf times to prevent crowding and ease beach access.

Tennis

Play outdoor tennis during daylight hours in order to prevent the need for energy-intensive nighttime lighting. Lighting for a single tennis court can consume more than 4,700 kilowatt-hours of energy per year, enough to power the average household for about six months.

" I've always been conscious about being healthy; as a professional athlete, I had to be. Being healthy means eating right and exercising and, in general, just doing what's right to stay in shape. But it also can be good for the planet: The healthier you eat, the less you consume foods that have pesticides and chemicals and things that create a lot of toxic waste when they're produced. Take fruits and vegetables. Just by choosing certain organic kinds, you can lower your exposure to pesticides. Exercising, too, is good for the planet: The more time you spend running, biking, swimming, lifting weights, or whatever, the less time you are likely using something that consumes energy, like your car or television.

By staying healthy yourself, you can keep the planet in good shape. "

money and finance

Money Makes the World Go 'Round

THE BIG PICTURE

Visits to the bank result in one of the biggest sources of litter on the planet: ATM receipts are tossed about as much as gum wrappers. With eight billion ATM transactions in the United States doling out $600 billion in cash per year, that's a lot of money to make the world go 'round. Unfortunately, the planet is paying for all those withdrawals by enduring the paper waste that is produced.

Still, people use paper checks, too, about thirty-seven billion of them a year. That's even more paper waste from banking. People use them to pay bills, mostly credit card bills. The average family in the United States has four credit cards. In total, that means there are about four hundred million little plastic cards in circulation in this country. Placed one in front of the other, they would forge a path more than twenty-one thousand miles long.

But it isn't so much the plastic waste that is a problem. Every month, a statement comes in the mail to go along with all those cards. Sometimes the statement is just a page. But in high spending season—such as, say, December—statements can be several pages long. The cost of paper processing is huge. However, bills aren't the only painful mailbox reminders of our finances. Taxes add up, too. When you're feeling blue about being in the red, think about this: General Electric's annual tax return amounts to almost 25,000 pages. Even if every U.S. taxpayer filed just a two-page 1040 EZ form, the total would add up to 270 million pages.

But all that paper waste pales in comparison with the amount of money that changes hands. About nineteen billion shares of stock trade every day around the world. Imagine if all the money invested went toward good causes, such as to companies that cared about protecting the planet. With $20 trillion worth of stock to choose from, investors can make a green statement by choosing to invest in socially responsible companies.

Keeping all that in mind, we've created the "Simple Steps" to be just that. Taking into account all the points of the Big Picture, they give you the biggest impact with the least amount of effort.

The Simple Steps

1. **Don't take an ATM receipt.** ATM receipts are one of the top sources of litter on the planet. If everyone in the United States left their receipt in the machine, it would save a roll of paper more than two billion feet long, or enough to circle the equator fifteen times.

2. **Request automatic deposits for your paychecks.** Not only will you get your money faster, but you'll reduce the time and fuel you spend to go to the bank. More than seven billion checks are written annually that could be replaced by automated deposits. If everyone who was eligible for an automated deposit opted for it, it would save about $65 billion in fuel costs and lost time expense—and enough paper checks for everyone in the world.

3. **Get paperless bank statements.** Some banks will pay you a dollar or donate the money on your behalf when you cancel the

monthly paper statements you get in the mail. If every household took advantage of online bank statements, the money saved could send more than seventeen thousand recent high school graduates to a public university for a year.

THE LITTLE THINGS

Advisers

Find one who is socially conscious. There are about six hundred thousand stockbrokers in the country, but only between one thousand and two thousand who say they invest with the environment in mind. Find one, and encourage more to think green.

Brokerage Statements

Go paperless. If every investor in the United States received paperless brokerage statements, it would save enough paper to fill the New York Stock Exchange from floor to ceiling.   .

Checks

Use electronic checks instead of paper checks. You'll save time and maybe even avoid late penalties! If everyone who uses paper checks made electronic payments instead, it would save about $4 billion in paper costs alone—enough to vaccinate every child in the United States against serious childhood diseases with all recommended vaccines.

Electronic Payments

Pay your bills electronically. If every household paid just its credit card bills electronically, it would save almost $2 billion a year in postage costs, or enough to wipe out average credit card debt for 250,000 people.

Electronic Tax Refunds

Take advantage of getting your money back electronically from the IRS instead of waiting for a check to arrive in the mail. About $135 billion in tax refunds still makes its way through the mail to individuals, which means the IRS has to stuff, print, and mail some fifty-four million envelopes.

Online Banking

Receive your bills, make payments, and check your account balance online. Less than half of all U.S. households use online banking capabilities at their home. Instead, they waste time and energy driving and waiting in line for the bank teller.

Paperless Accounting

Try reconciling your bills with software rather than a paper check register. If every household used paperless accounting for record keeping rather than their manual checkbook ledger, they would save enough paper for a check big enough to cover (literally) all the office space used by both the Department of the Treasury and the U.S. Federal Reserve, including all of its banks.

Prospectuses

Read investment prospectuses online rather than in book form. (You'll likely get one from any mutual fund in which you invest.) It's easier to scan online for important information than flipping through pages. If every investor chose this option, the savings in printing costs would total $1 billion—enough money to rank 374th on the Forbes 400 list of wealthiest people—and would save hundreds of millions more in pages of paper.

Proxy Statements

Request electronic delivery of proxies. When shareholders try to change the way a corporation acts, they issue proxy statements to get others to vote along with them—sometimes even to pressure a company to be more environmentally friendly. It's easier to vote online, however, and saves $600 million a year in printing costs—or about how much Enron overstated its earnings.

Socially Responsible Investing

Try to buy more environmentally friendly stocks and products. There are more than two hundred mutual funds—out of some eight thousand mutual funds in total—that are socially and environmentally conscious.

Stock Certificates

Request that stock certificates of ownership be held in your brokerage firm's name instead of your own. (When you buy stock in a company, you are entitled to a certificate of ownership.) Having your brokerage hold these saves having mostly useless paper certificates sent to you.

Tax Forms

Get your tax forms online. It's simpler, and you can file faster. Over seventy-two million tax returns are e-filed, twenty million from home computers. If every tax return were e-filed, it would save at least 660 million sheets of paper—stacked to equal more than thirty-six thousand six-foot-tall IRS agents.

Trade Confirmations

Don't ask for your trade confirmations. When you buy and/or sell stock, a confirmation of the transaction can be sent to you. Instead, have confirms e-mailed. Twenty billion shares of stock trade daily. If we could eliminate the dollar cost of paper processing trade confirmations alone, and instead used that money for another purpose, we could cut by half the number of people living in poverty throughout the world—in one day.

Withdrawals/Deposits

Don't take a slip. Use an ATM rather than a bank teller. The cost of an ATM transaction is thirty-six cents, whereas it costs more than a dollar to process a transaction through a branch teller, who has to use and process more paper. If every bank teller in the United States handled one less deposit slip per hour, at least four million pieces of paper could be saved per day.

"I started driving a Prius a few years ago, and I was surprised to find myself a little defensive about it.

'You know, aside from the whole environmental thing,' I'd say, almost dismissively, 'it's actually a pretty cool car to drive.' It was like I was halfway apologetic because I didn't want to be aligned with any group, or movement. Sort of like, 'Hey, just because I'm driving a hybrid doesn't mean I'm turning into Ed Begley Jr.'

But you know how people say marijuana is a gateway drug? That's sorta what buying a Prius was for me . . . in terms of becoming environmentally sensitive. Because before too long, I stopped wondering if driving it made me some kind of a preachy do-gooder, and I actually started looking for other ways to 'go green.'

Organic food was an easy one: I always liked the idea of eating healthy, just never did it much. But I do now, and it makes me feel better. I started using paper towels that aren't really paper towels (well, they are, but somehow they are recycled), and cleaning supplies that maybe don't clean completely as good as the old stuff—but they also don't leave your house with that weird, slightly toxic smell. And then I read that you could get solar panels put on your house, and that they pay for themselves over time (a long, long, long time); and I have those now.

I've even started worrying about my carbon footprint—for starters, what is a carbon footprint?—and it occurred to me the other day that, dammit, I AM Ed Begley Jr., or I'd like to be . . . because I love this planet, and I love nature, and I love taking walks on the beach at sunset. And if that makes me sound like Miss February filling out her turn-ons in a *Playboy* bio, so be it."

building

If We Build It Green, They Will Come

THE BIG PICTURE

More than a million or so new homes are built in the United States each year. That's an awful lot of wood, metal, and concrete being put to use, never mind all the digging and hammering. In fact, the use of the land and wood alone for new-home construction is responsible for about a quarter of our total impact on wildlife and natural ecosystems. Think about the size of the effect when you add in the production of steel beams, cement foundations, tile, carpet, stucco, windows, and insulation. Six percent of water pollution comes from manufacturing the materials for new homes, and in terms of energy, it's huge: You can live in your home for ten years before you will use the amount of energy it took to make it.

The issue isn't just the number of homes being built; it's also that homes are getting bigger. The average size of a new home in the United States has increased from 1,500 square feet in 1970 to about 2,300 square feet today, while the average family size has decreased from more than three people to a little more than two people. The average

U.S. home is now twice the size of the typical home in Europe or Japan and twenty-six times larger than the average living space in Africa.

What's all this extra space used for? Playrooms. Media rooms. Workrooms. Sitting rooms. Laundry rooms. Libraries. Sunrooms. Larger kitchens. Bigger bathrooms. His and her closets. And more. No matter the purpose of the space, energy is consumed to keep temperatures comfortable, rooms well lit, electronic gadgets working, and appliances humming along. The tab for all this adds up to about $1,500 a year. But it doesn't have to add up that way.

About 80 percent of new homes built are not energy efficient, when they could easily be.

They could also be more water efficient. The typical household wastes about eight thousand gallons a year just waiting for hot water to arrive at the tap. Watering the lawns in America claims an estimated eight billion gallons of water—a volume that would fill fourteen billion six-packs of beer. During summer, the average lawn uses about ten thousand gallons of water!

Even a home's position against the sun and wind has ramifications that can add 25 percent to its heating bill. And it goes the other way, too: The total amount of energy lost through windows in the United States each year is equivalent to the annual energy output of the Alaska oil pipeline.

Keeping all that in mind, we've created the "Simple Steps" to be just that. Taking into account all the points of the Big Picture, they give you the biggest impact with the least amount of effort.

The Simple Steps

1. **Buy Energy Star appliances and electronics.** Households that use Energy Star products automatically become more energy efficient and can save $600 a year in energy costs. In 2005 alone, Energy Star helped Americans reduce their greenhouse gas emissions by an amount equivalent to those from twenty-three million cars and save enough on their energy bills to buy every product sold on eBay for three straight months.

2. **Install low-flow plumbing.** An average three-member household can reduce its water consumption by fifty-four thousand gallons annually and can lower its water bills by about $60 per year if water-efficient plumbing fixtures are used. If every U.S. household used low-flow plumbing fixtures, it would save $6 billion, or enough to buy a bottle of water for everyone on the planet.

3. **Get ceiling fans and use them instead of air-conditioning.** It costs just a penny an hour to run a ceiling fan versus sixteen cents an hour for a room air conditioner and forty-three cents an hour for central air. More than 75 percent of U.S. households use air-conditioning and in doing so waste $12 million per hour in energy costs when ceiling fans would do.

THE LITTLE THINGS

Absorbent Materials

For patios, paths, and walkways, consider laying gravel, wood chips, nutshells, or other salvaged materials that encourage water to seep back into the ground. Depending on your local climate, you could reduce runoff from your property by several thousand gallons per year and prevent certain types of water pollution.

Adhesives

Adhesives used for flooring, cabinetry, and furniture can often contain more hazardous chemicals than the materials they are bonding. For that reason, it's best to employ installation techniques that avoid the use of adhesives whenever possible. If adhesives are required for your project, try to select brands that are water or vegetable based. You'll reduce hazardous emissions by over 99 percent compared with adhesives that contain petroleum-derived solvents.

Air-Conditioning

Buy an Energy Star system. The average home owner spends over $220 per year on air-conditioning. Energy Star–labeled air conditioners will use 20 to 40 percent less energy than standard systems. If all new homes were equipped with Energy Star air conditioners, it could save as much as former presidents Bush and Clinton raised for Hurricane Katrina relief, about $100 million.

Bathroom Countertops

If you're planning to buy a hard-surface plastic bathroom countertop, consider one made from 100 percent recycled materials. You'll prevent about forty pounds of plastic from being landfilled. If one out of every ten bathrooms remodeled this year were furnished with a recycled plastic countertop, twenty million pounds of plastic could be diverted from the waste stream, or the equivalent in weight of about four million plastic toilet seats.

Carpet

Instead of buying carpet made from synthetic fibers, you can save manufacturing energy, reduce toxic emissions, and close the recycling loop by choosing carpet produced from recycled materials such as plastic bottles. If you recarpet 1,500 square feet of your home with recycled-content carpet, you could prevent the equivalent of more than eight thousand two-liter bottles from being landfilled. If you applied this to just 13 percent of new carpeting installed, the equivalent of nearly twelve billion two-liter bottles could be saved. Stood upright, side by side, they'd cover an area the size of Boston.

Cooling/Heating Systems

Install programmable thermostats for your heating and cooling systems. A programmable thermostat can save you about $100 every year in energy costs. If just one in ten households did this, we'd prevent seventeen billion pounds of greenhouse gases from being let loose, or about as much gas as all the cows in the United States burp per day! Cows burp methane, a greenhouse gas.

Create an Envelope

You can create an improved envelope of insulation around your home by building with materials that reduce drafts and by sealing cracks and gaps that permit air and moisture exchanges. This could reduce your heating and cooling costs by about 2,250 kilowatt-hours of energy and $180 per year. If every new home were built with a tightly insulated envelope, the energy savings would equate to more than doubling the fuel efficiency of the 210,000 postal vehicles that deliver the U.S. mail.

Drywall

Try to find drywall made with at least 75 percent recycled content, including 10 percent or greater postconsumer content. You may also consider drywall produced with synthetic gypsum or fly ash instead of natural gypsum. In both cases, you'll help save energy, reduce waste, and reduce the habitat disruption associated with gypsum mining. If just 1 percent of all drywall used for U.S. construction each year had at least 75 percent recycled content, the total materials saved could build a sheet of drywall nearly eleven feet high and as long as the Great Wall of China.

Dual-Flush Toilets

Buy them and save water. They come with two flush options: The first uses 0.8 gallons of water, and the second uses 1.6 gallons (to dispose of more waste). This can reduce water usage by up to 67 percent compared with the traditional toilet, which uses about 3 gallons in a single flush. If every household had a dual-flush toilet, the total savings from a single flush per home would equal the amount of water flushed in stadium bathrooms throughout the entire baseball season.

Erosion/Sedimentation

Limit vegetation removal during your home's construction to help prevent erosion. Erosion is a leading source of pollution to America's rivers, lakes, and streams because home drainage and storm water runoff contain harmful chemicals.

Fabrics

Choose recycled fabrics for couches, drapes, chairs, and other upholstery. If half of the polyester fabric made in the United States each year were produced with recycled materials, it would be enough to cover the entire state of New York.

Finishes

You can avoid harmful toxins, air-polluting chemicals, and petroleum solvents by purchasing varnishes, stains, and finishes that contain low or no volatile organic compounds (VOCs). VOCs are main contributors to smog, and the amount saved by choosing a few gallons of low-VOC coating is roughly the amount of VOC you'd save if you avoided driving your car for an entire year. If half of all wood flooring installed per year were coated with low-VOC products, the effect would be equivalent to eliminating the annual VOC emissions from nearly two hundred thousand cars.

Furniture

Your best option for furniture is to buy used, refurbished, or antique items. Not only may you pay a lower price than you would for new furniture, but you'll conserve manufacturing energy and materials and prevent vintage pieces from being tossed into landfills. Across America, an increase in demand for used furniture would help reduce the more than seventeen billion pounds of furniture that are tossed into landfills every year. If you can't find vintage furniture you like, try to buy furniture made from sustainably produced materials, such as plantation-grown lumber or wood certified by the Forest Stewardship Council. Try to avoid furniture made from certain hardwoods, such as teak, mahogany, rosewood, and hemlock. Harvesting these species contributes greatly to tropical deforestation, an annual loss of rain forest area larger than the state of Alabama.

Garage

Build a detached garage, or make sure it's sealed off from the rest of the house, and you'll improve air quality. Indoor air pollution makes you sick. Air quality problems cost U.S. businesses 150 million workdays and about $15 billion in productivity losses each year.

Glass Tiles

Instead of buying ceramic tiles for countertops, backsplashes, or flooring, choose 100 percent recycled glass tiles. For every one hundred square feet of recycled glass tiles that replace traditional ceramic tiles, 140 kilowatt-hours of manufacturing energy are conserved. This is roughly the amount of energy that your refrigerator uses per month. If an additional 15 percent of tiles purchased per year were made from recycled glass instead of ceramic material, the total energy saved could allow for the shutdown of five highly polluting coal-fired power plants.

Greenfields vs. Brownfields

Instead of constructing a new home or business on "new" land (green-fields), consider building on sites that may have infrastructure already in place (brownfields). You'll help reduce urban sprawl; preserve watersheds, native landscapes, fish, and wildlife habitats; and may qualify for a tax credit as well. If all new development occurring on greenfields were instead reallocated to brownfields, more than two million acres of open space could be preserved annually.

Hardwood Flooring

Select bamboo as an attractive, affordable, and sustainable alternative to conventionally harvested hardwood floors and you'll save three "old growth" trees—trees that may have started growing before your grandparents were born. Bamboo regenerates in less than seven years, so it can be continually harvested. If every hardwood floor purchased this year—nearly one billion square feet—were substituted with one made from bamboo, the volume of wood saved could provide every U.S. city, town, village, and borough with its own eight-acre forest of old-growth trees.

Highly Reflective Roofing

If you're building a new home or installing a new roof, select highly reflective roofing material. You could save an average of 1,100 kilowatt-hours of energy and $90 per year in cooling costs—more than you'd conserve by adjusting your thermostat by three degrees. If one in sixty-six new homes were covered with highly reflective roofs, the total energy saved would be equivalent to the amount generated by a solar panel roof the size of the Pentagon.

Insulated Wall Panels

As an alternative to traditional wood framing, consider building with insulated concrete wall panels. Since these panels offer better temperature regulation during both warm and cool seasons, you may reduce your annual energy consumption by an average of roughly one thousand kilowatt-hours and $80 per year. If 1 percent of new-home construction this year used insulated wall panels, the annual energy savings would equal 2,137 tons of coal—enough to build a wall of coal ten feet high and nearly a mile long.

Insulation

For both new and existing homes, choose insulation made from recycled newspaper, glass, or other recovered materials. The energy required to manufacture recycled insulation is less than one-sixth that needed to produce fiberglass insulation. If every new home built in the United States this year were insulated with recycled content insulation, the total manufacturing energy saved could heat and cool thirty-five thousand housing units for the next seventeen years.

Kitchen Countertops

If you choose a durable composite, paper stone, terrazzo, stainless-steel, or tile countertop with 50 to 100 percent recycled content, you'll reduce the manufacturing energy and waste associated with producing new materials. However, since few countertops are recyclable (with the exception of stainless steel), the best thing you can do for the environment is to choose a long-lasting countertop that will survive the average ten-year remodeling itch. If every new countertop installed this year could be made to last twice as long, the savings could build a 2.5-foot-wide countertop that stretched from the North Pole to Antarctica.

Landscaping

Keep your grounds planted with what grows naturally in your area. Natural landscapes do not require mowing, whereas lawns must be mowed regularly. Gas-powered garden tools emit 5 percent of the nation's air pollution, as they use some six hundred million gallons of gasoline per year. One gas-powered lawn mower emits eleven times more air pollution than the average new car for each hour of operation.

Lighting

Install more efficient lighting systems, such as those with motion sensors and dimmable lighting controls. And, of course, go fluorescent. You can save $35 annually if you replace just four standard incandescent lamps with compact fluorescent lamps, which use 66 percent less energy. If every American home replaced just one light bulb with a more energy-efficient one, we would save enough energy to light more than 2.5 million homes for a year and prevent greenhouse gases equivalent to the emissions of nearly eight hundred thousand cars.

Linoleum vs. Vinyl

Linoleum is made from all-natural resources, while vinyl flooring is made from petroleum-derived plastic. If instead of installing a five-hundred-square-foot vinyl floor you chose a linoleum one, you could save the energy equivalent of twelve gallons of gasoline. If just 1 percent of the hard-surface flooring sold in the United States per year were linoleum instead of vinyl, the oil saved would equal six hundred thousand barrels—nearly as much as the United States imports daily from Iraq.

Natural Site Features

Take into consideration the natural landscape when you build, and you can save on construction costs. Sustainable building sites reduce costs for site preparation, infrastructure construction, and infrastructure maintenance, especially for storm water, which can be managed using the natural landscape. This can add up to a 20 percent savings and helps prevent future maintenance costs.

Orientation

You could save significant energy by selecting a house where most of the windows face north or south. Try to avoid building or buying a home with most of its windows facing west, as these will receive direct sunlight during the hottest part of the day and could raise your cooling bills by 25 percent.

Paint

For every gallon of 100 percent recycled paint purchased, you'll prevent a gallon of paint from being tossed into a toxic waste dump. Recycled paint usually costs an average of 30 to 50 percent less than a gallon of virgin paint. If one in fifteen new gallons of paint purchased were 100 percent recycled, the total paint savings would equal forty million gallons—enough to give every paved road in California a coat of royal blue. If recycled paint is unavailable, choose latex paint over oil based, especially for interior uses. It releases fewer toxins, contains fewer petrochemicals, and is easier to dispose of.

Porous Pavement

Consider using porous pavement instead of asphalt for driveways. Porous pavement prevents unnatural water runoff, reduces drainage problems, and helps keep pollutants from entering groundwater. If all of the asphalt parking lots and driveways in the United States were replaced by porous paving, there would be enough asphalt to make a parking lot the size of South Dakota.

Roof

Use light-colored roofing made from recycled materials. You'll lower the "heat island" effect of your home, keeping it cooler in the summer. Ninety percent of the roofs in the United States are dark colored. A cooler roof means savings on summertime air-conditioning (up to $34 per one thousand square feet of roof), reducing the demand for electrical power and lowering air pollution and greenhouse gas emissions.

Shade

You could reduce your annual cooling costs by up to 25 percent by building extended eaves, planting leafy trees, constructing an arbor, or installing awnings to shade the south or west faces of your home. For the average home, the savings could equal seven hundred kilowatt-hours per year of energy, or roughly $56. Across 5 percent of owner-occupied homes in the United States, the annual energy savings from increased shade could total nearly two billion kilowatt-hours of energy—enough to fly nearly every resident of Phoenix to the shady beaches of the Sunshine State.

Site Selection

Select a home site that will minimize your travel distances and time to work, schools, shopping, and the like. If you built your home at a site that was just one mile closer to where you work, you'd commute an average of five hundred fewer miles per year, saving about 20 gallons of gasoline. If one in ten new-home buyers selected a home site that cut his or her commute by one mile each way, 2.4 million gallons of gas could be saved per year—enough to fuel more than ten thousand road trips between Los Angeles and New York City.

Slopes

If you're planning to build on a sloped site, you can reduce the effects of erosion as well as save money and energy by locating your structure on the least sloped portion of the lot. The grading of slopes to achieve a level site results in excessive topsoil loss, sedimentation, and water pollution. Also, the use of earth-moving equipment is both energy intensive and expensive. In all cases, try to avoid the disturbance of steep slopes by maintaining natural hillside vegetation, building runoff catchments, and landscaping with native shrubs, trees, and ground cover.

Soil

Stockpile the topsoil that is removed for foundation laying during your home construction and then reapply it to areas that will be landscaped once your home is built. You'll conserve the energy and money that would be spent to transport this soil to a recycling location or landfill. If you need more soil, use or purchase 100 percent recycled compost or mulch.

Solar

Install solar panels and get free energy from the sun. Solar panels may be costly to install, but they pay for themselves after about ten years with rebates and tax credits. Each day, more solar energy falls to the earth than the total amount of energy the planet's 6.6 billion human inhabitants would consume in twenty-seven years. Currently, we harness only about 1 percent of the sun's energy.

Solar Water Heaters

Look into installing a solar water heater. You may be able to save $450 per year in energy costs. Solar water heaters cost more to purchase and install, but the energy savings and tax credits can pay for the difference in just three years. If solar collectors heated the twenty-five gallons or so of hot water that each person uses per day, the sun's free energy would save us $135 billion a year.

Treated Wood

As an alternative to treated wood for decks, landscaping, or benches, choose recycled plastic lumber. You'll prevent the leaching of toxic chemicals from treated wood into soil and water supplies, save trees, and remove plastic from the waste stream. An eight-by-ten-foot deck made with 50 percent recycled plastic lumber would save the equivalent of about 1,700 plastic milk jugs from being discarded at landfills. If just 1 percent of the treated wood purchased for residential decks each year were replaced with recycled plastic lumber, the total savings could equal more than 1 billion plastic jugs and one thousand acres of redwood forest.

Trees

You could save over 20 percent on your air-conditioning bill per year by planting two twenty-five-foot shade trees on the west and one on the east side of your home. If shade trees were planted around just 25 percent of dwellings with air-conditioning, the energy savings would be enough to shut down three coal-fired power plants.

Windbreaks

You can protect your home from the effects of cold winter winds by planting a windbreak—a dense row of evergreen shrubs and small trees—along the north or west side of your house. The height of your windbreak should be about one-half to one-fifth the distance from your house to where your windbreak is planted (if you wanted to plant a windbreak thirty feet away from your home, the trees and shrubs should be about fifteen feet tall). A windbreak could reduce your annual heating energy costs by over 1,400 kilowatt-hours and $110. If one in ten rural households planted a windbreak, the energy savings could meet the heating oil needs of more than fifty-seven thousand Alaskan homes for an entire year.

Windows

Get double-pane windows, and buy according to your climate. This can save up to $400 a year in energy costs. If every household saved this much by installing more energy-efficient windows, it would keep $110 million per day in energy costs from going out the window.

Wood

If you're building a new home, you'll save roughly eighty-eight trees, or 3.2 acres of forest, by choosing recycled wood. Since most recycled wood was originally derived from old-growth trees, it is of higher quality than standard lumber. As such, it can be four times more energy efficient and will last three to four times as long. If one in six new homes used recycled lumber, a forest larger than Yosemite National Park could be preserved every year. If recycled wood is not available from your local lumberyard, try to purchase wood that has been certified by the Forest Stewardship Council. You'll ensure that the wood you buy was harvested in a sustainable manner—not harming fragile habitats, water supplies, or indigenous communities. Currently, more than 115 million acres of forest in sixty-one countries have received certification by the Forest Stewardship Council.

"The trip that I recently took to Africa was really an eye-opening experience for me. It led me to this place, a place I hadn't thought about before in my mind. You see so many things and you want to help. It's an education.

We met a group of kids being educated on HIV, some people my age. Over here, we learn about some of that stuff in the fifth and sixth grade!

A lot of things like that stuck with me, because there are so many problems and so many people who need help. And it all goes back to the environment, and our relationship to it, and what we can do to help ourselves.

Water is such a huge issue, and food. Then you think about where that all comes from. Then you think about sanitation and how that can lead to disease. Like I said, there's so much.

I wanted to save the world in the palm of my hand. Anyone with half a heart who sees the statistics would want to do as much as they could and contribute as much as they can. But you realize that it's a marathon, not a sprint. So I wanted to do what would be most effective with my time and my energy.

I was working on this album at the time, and I knew I was going to be putting a tour together for it, so it just made a lot of sense to think about carbon offsetting. It all just coincided with my schedule.

I hadn't really thought about how much you emit on tour, how much all those trucks emit. In your mind, you simply don't think about all that pollution. So here I am going on tour, and I'm thinking carbon offsetting is going to make a huge dent in my footprint; I am going on tour for a whole year.

It's what I can do right now."

going carbon neutral

Greentag, You're It

THE BIG PICTURE

Global warming is real. The average temperature of the earth's atmosphere has increased by one degree Fahrenheit in recent decades. And just that little amount is having a huge effect on the planet: Ice caps melt, seas rise, floods ensue. Global warming can even heighten the intensity of storms and weather patterns.

Global warming works like this: The sun heats the earth's atmosphere every day. That heat hits the earth's surface and bounces back into outer space. But some of that heat is trapped, which is good because without it, well, think Ice Age. Global warming becomes a problem when too much of that heat remains in the atmosphere. Now think scorching hot desert.

One of the main elements that traps more heat within the earth's atmosphere is carbon—specifically in the form of carbon dioxide. And that's because of us and all our activities. When oil, coal, gasoline, or natural gas is burned, carbon is released into the atmosphere. So when we run our cars, light and heat our homes, and manufacture our goods, we emit more carbon. You don't have to be a scientist to recognize that since the dawn of man we have been doing more and more of this.

Trees come into the picture because they suck up carbon and turn it into oxygen for us. But as we chop down more trees to make paper and wood products such as furniture and building materials, and clear forests to raise livestock, we have less and less "natural" help removing carbon from the air.

Now this is where we come in. We can reduce the amount of carbon we release into the atmosphere by following some of the tips in this book. Or we can take it a step further and "offset" our own carbon emissions.

We can offset the amount of carbon each of us is responsible for by purchasing carbon credits. These credits go toward planting more trees to suck up the carbon each of us uses or to fund "clean energy"—like wind and solar power—that doesn't produce carbon. The more we rely on clean energy, the less we'll rely on energy that produces carbon. Scientists have developed methods to calculate the amount of carbon each of us uses in our daily lives. And once we compute that individual contribution of carbon, we can choose ways to offset it.

It works like this: You take the amount of carbon you produce by, say, driving your car. (See the following formula for how to calculate.) If you produce three hundred pounds of carbon dioxide a month by driving, you could choose to buy an equal amount of carbon certificates to offset your driving.

Carbon certificates are sold by firms that invest in clean energy projects. They pool all the money they receive and fund more tree planting, or solar-powered energy plants, or wind farms. Airlines are starting to offer the option of carbon-offsetting trips to passengers, as are other companies that use lots of carbon-emitting energy. Carbon-offsetting firms can be easily found on the Internet.

Carbon offsetting, sometimes called "going carbon neutral" or "greentagging," is important for the following reason: If ice shelves keep melting at their current rate, cities like Los Angeles, New York, Miami, New Orleans, and London will become completely submerged, not to mention the hundreds of other coastal cities around the world.

Droughts will occur inland, and food and water shortages will follow. Wildfires will increase, plants and animals will die. Diseases will increase as people are forced to live closer together, and there will be fewer natural resources to go around. The planet will literally begin to die.

It sounds like the makings of a science fiction movie, but it isn't. It is the ultimate big-picture problem we are facing today.

Carbon offsetting takes more effort than a simple shift in habit, and it costs money. Sometimes not a lot, but as we've seen, little things can add up.

Keeping all this in mind, we've created the "Simple Steps" to be just that. Taking into account all the points of the Big Picture, they allow you to make the biggest positive planetary impact with the least amount of effort.

The Simple Steps

1. **Carbon offset your air travel.** Every passenger mile you fly emits 0.64 pound of carbon dioxide. So if you fly about 3,100 miles round trip across the country, multiply that by 0.64 to get approximately one ton of carbon dioxide as your total contribution to carbon emissions.

Flight Miles per Year _____ (× 0.64) = Year Total _____

2. **Carbon offset your driving.** If you have a small car, figure you may get as much as twenty-nine miles per gallon. Every gallon of gas you use emits about twenty pounds of carbon dioxide. The average car gets about twenty miles per gallon—or about one pound per mile. The average American automobile's carbon footprint is estimated at six tons (twelve thousand pounds) of carbon dioxide annually. So if you do the math: Take the number of gallons you put in

your gas tank per month and multiply it by 20 to figure your carbon emissions from driving.

Car Miles per Year ____ (× 1.0) = Year Total ____

3. **Carbon offset your home energy use.** If you use electricity, you'll emit on average 1.34 pounds of carbon dioxide per kilowatt-hour. If you use natural gas, you'll emit on average 12.06 pounds of carbon dioxide per therm. If you use heating oil, you'll emit on average 22.38 pounds of carbon dioxide per gallon. And if you use propane, you'll emit 12.8 pounds of carbon dioxide per gallon.

Electricity per Year (kilowatt-hours) ____ (× 1.34) = Year Total ____
Natural Gas per Year (therms) ____ (× 12.06) = Year Total ____
Home Heating Oil per Year (gallons) ____ (× 22.38) = Year Total ____
Propane per Year (gallons) ____ (× 12.8) = Year Total ____

Grand Carbon Total ____

Once you've figured your total carbon emissions, it will be easy to offset your energy footprint by purchasing the appropriate amount of carbon credits. Carbon credits are sold on a per ton basis at approximately $12 per ton (one short ton = two thousand pounds).

To reduce your carbon footprint and therefore save on the amount of carbon credits you'll need to offset your emissions, you can also try some of the following suggestions:

THE LITTLE THINGS

Air Conditioner

Tune up your air conditioner and you could save 220 pounds of carbon and $14 per year.

Auto
Switch to a more fuel-efficient car. Every mile per gallon gained reduces your carbon emission by one pound.

Free Transportation
Walk or bike and create zero carbon emissions from fossil fuels.

Furnace
Tune up your furnace and you could save 335 pounds of carbon per year. For gas, you could save 252 pounds per year.

Insulation
Insulate your doors and windows with weather stripping and you could save on electricity 1,600 pounds of carbon and $100 per year, on oil 1,000 pounds of carbon per year, and on gas 700 pounds of carbon per year.

Put an insulation jacket around your home water heater and you could save on electricity 600 pounds of carbon and $38 per year, on oil 360 pounds per year, and on gas 260 pounds of carbon per year.

Light Bulbs
Replace conventional incandescent light bulbs with compact fluorescent light bulbs in your home (twenty-seven-watt compact fluorescent bulbs replace seventy-five-watt incandescent bulbs; eighteen-watt fluorescent bulbs replace sixty-watt incandescent bulbs). For each twenty-seven-watt compact fluorescent light bulb you'll get carbon emissions savings of 140 pounds per year and save $12.00. For each eighteen-watt compact fluorescent light bulb, you'll get carbon emission savings of 110 pounds per year and save $9.50.

Public Transportation
Take a bus. A bus emits about 2.75 pounds of carbon per mile; divided by the number of passengers on it, however, this can create carbon savings.

Recycle

Recycling saves, too: Every ten aluminum or steel cans recycled saves four pounds of carbon, and every ten glass bottles recycled saves three pounds carbon. If you recycle newspapers, you could save fifty pounds of carbon per year.

Thermostat

Turn down your thermostat at night. For each degree, you save about 1 percent on your heating costs and carbon emissions. If you turn down the heat in your home overnight or when no one is home—for argument's sake, half the day—by ten degrees, you can save about 10 percent.

The goal, of course, is to get as close to zero carbon emissions as possible.

If we all did it: We'd save the planet.

references

The Big Picture
http://www.iwmi.cgiar.org/home/wsmap.htm
http://www.eia.doe.gov/kids/energyfacts/uses/consumption.html

The Simple Steps
SHORTER SHOWER
http://www.monolake.org/socalwater/wctips.htm
http://www.ocf.berkeley.edu/~sgb/pledge/pledgeinfo/26%20showers.doc
http://www.consumerreports.org/cro/personal-finance/50-ways-to-save-water-805/
    index.htm
http://www.apexnc.org/depts/pw/water_cons.cfm
http://www.aga.wisc.edu.waterlibrary/facts.asp

ADJUST THERMOSTAT
http://www.robhogg.org/content.asp?ID=1932&I=4920
http://www.energystar.gov

RECYCLING
http://www.answers.com/topic/scrap-and-waste-materials

The Little Things
IN THE KITCHEN
Composting
http://www.epa.gov/epaoswer/non-hw/composting/index.htm
http://wastec.isproductions.net/webmodules/webarticles/anmviewer.asp?a=1123
http://onlineconversion.com/area.htm
http://quickfacts.census.gov/qfd/states/06/0667000.html

Dishwasher
http://www.ci.greeley.co.us/cog/PageServiceDetails.asp?fkOrgID=44&SDID=1
http://www.consumerreports.org/cro/personal-finance/50-ways-to-save-water-805/
    index.htm

http://www.conservewater.utah.gov/IndoorUse/Kitchen/
http://www.we-energies.com/residential/energyeff/101tips.htm#refrig
http://www.leeric.lsu.edu/energy/hot_water/#insulate

Food Waste
http://www.catalystmagazine.net/issues/story.cfm?story=1042
http://starbulletin.com/2001/12/08/news/whatever.html
http://www.nationalhomeless.org/publications/facts/education.pdf

Garbage Disposal
http://www.city-of-torrington.org/water_wise_page.htm
http://www.bigjonseptic.com/
http://www.grinningplanet.com/2005/05-10/sink-garbage-disposal-problems-odor-
   article.htm
http://www.miamidade.gov/derm/tips/tips_garbage_disposal.asp

Microwave
http://www.unep.org/geo2000/english/i5a.htm
http://www.energyhawk.com/cooking/cooking3.php
http://www.aps.com/images/pdf/Cooking.pdf

Preheating
http://www.p2pays.org/ref/14/13105.pdf
http://www.bostonapartments.com/enrgyapt.htm
http://www.msichicago.org/ed/coal/coalcalc.html

Refrigerator
http://www.mbm.net.au/uss/check_list.html
http://www.energystar.gov/index.cfm?c=about.ab_index
http://www.weenergies.com/residential/energyeff/101tips.htm#refrig
http://www.worldwise.com/reffreez.html
http://www.state.co.us/oemc/publications/Home_Energy_Saving_Tips.htm

Storage Containers
http://www.grinningplanet.com/2004/11-09/chemicals-plastic-storage-containers-
   article.htm
http://www.treehugger.com/files/interiors/storage/

Stove
http://www.unu.edu/unupress/food/8F072e/8F072E06.htm
http://www.energystar.gov/index.cfm?c=products.es_at_home_tips
http://www.eartheasy.com/live_energyeffic_appl.htm
http://www.wrec.net/energytips.htm

Trash Bags
http://www.albertsons.com/store/?market=11
http://www.sierraclub.org/bags/

Water Filters
http://www.allaboutwater.org/water-filter.html
http://www.advancedwaterfilters.com/whole-house-water-filter.html

IN THE BATHROOM
Brushing Your Teeth
http://www.ocf.berkeley.edu/~sgb/pledge/pledgeinfo/27%20brush%20shave.doc
http://www.consumerreports.org/cro/personal-finance/50-ways-to-save-water-805/
    index.htm
http://www.charlottesville.org/Index.aspx?page=640
http://www.gru.com/YourHome/Conservation/Water/waterSavers.jsp
http://www.gothamgazette.com/article/20031208/200/796

Shaving
http://www.ocf.berkeley.edu/~sgb/pledge/pledgeinfo/27%20brush%20shave.doc
http://www.downers.us/pubworks/water/div/inwaterconserve.htm
http://www.fi.edu/weather/drought.html
http://www.americanwater.com/49ways.htm

Shower Curtains
http://www.eia.doe.gov/kids/energyfacts/saving/recycling/solidwaste/plastics.html
http://www.treehugger.com/files/2005/09/qa_non-vinyl_sh.php
http://www.rawganique.com/BAsc1.htm
http://www.ecobathroom.com/shop/hempshowercurtain.html

Toilet
http://www.consumerreports.org/cro/personal-finance/50-ways-to-save-water-805/
    index.htm
http://www.wateruseitwisely.com/100ways/sw.shtml
http://www.ocf.berkeley.edu/~sgb/pledge/pledgeinfo/26%20showers.doc
http://www.apexnc.org/depts/pw/water_cons.cfm
http://www.monolake.org/socalwater/wctips.htm

Tub
http://www.apexnc.org/depts/pw/water_cons.cfm
http://www.consumerreports.org/cro/personal-finance/50-ways-to-save-water-805/index.htm
http://www.wateruseitwisely.com/100ways/sw.shtml
http://www.epa.gov/OW/you/chap3.html
http://www.ocf.berkeley.edu/~sgb/pledge/pledgeinfo/26%20showers.doc
http://www.apexnc.org/depts/pw/water_cons.cfm
http://www.monolake.org/socalwater/wctips.htm
http://www.statoids.com/yco.html
http://www.space.com/scienceastronomy/101_earth_facts_030722-3.html

IN THE LIVING ROOM
Fireplace
http://www.unu.edu/unupress/food/8F072e/8F072E06.htm
http://www.energyquest.ca.gov/saving_energy/index.html

http://www.siliconvalleypower.com/res/articles/?sub=fireplaces
http://www.lowes.com/lowes/lkn?action=howTo&p=Improve/HomeEnergyEfficient.html#8
http://www1.eere.energy.gov/consumer/tips/fireplaces.html

Junk Mail
http://www.stopjunkmail.org/resident2.htm
http://www.dmaconsumers.org/cgi/offmailing

Light Bulbs
http://www.vanityfair.com/
http://www.energystar.gov
http://www.powerhousetv.com/stellent2/groups/public/documents/pub/phtv_se_li_
    000566.hcsp
http://worldwise.stores.yahoo.net/lightbulbs.html
http://www.thefulcrumintl.com/Home/Article.aspx?article=185

Matches vs. Lighters
http://environment.guardian.co.uk/columnist/story/0,,1855171,00.html

Shades/Drapes
http://www.eia.doe.gov/kids/energyfacts/saving/efficiency/savingenergy.html
http://www.curtainandbath.com/energy_saving_items.htm
http://www.bpa.gov/Energy/n/Energy_Tips/save_energy/heating.cfm

IN THE UTILITY CLOSET
Air Conditioner and Furnace Filters
http://www.allergybuyersclubshopping.com/elguarfil.html#review
http://en.wikipedia.org/wiki/Washington,_D.C.

Dry Cleaning
http://www.bagbarn.com/garment.htm
http://www.sunnysideoflouisville.org/bureau/hotairballoon.htm

Dryers
http://www.eartheasy.com/live_energyeffic_appl.htm
http://www.leeric.lsu.edu/energy/hot_water/#insulate
http://www.consumerenergycenter.org/tips/summer.html
http://www.wrec.net/energytips.htm
http://www.everythingscool.org/downloads/EnergyTips_walletcard01.pdf

Phone Books
http://www.greenbiz.com/toolbox/essentials_third.cfm?LinkAdvID=4164
http://www.ci.amarillo.tx.us/pdf/City%20Notes%20April%202006.pdf

Washers
http://www.eartheasy.com/live_energyeffic_appl.htm
http://www.consumerenergycenter.org/tips/summer.html

http://www.wrec.net/energytips.htm
http://www.leeric.lsu.edu/energy/hot_water/#insulate

Water Heaters
http://www.stopglobalwarming.org/sgw_actionitems.asp
http://www.wrec.net/energytips.htm

IN THE GARAGE
Car Idling
http://maine.sierraclub.org/cap_join.htm
http://www.offroaders.com/tech/healthier-garage.htm
http://www.unc.edu/~awise/My%20Webs/garage1.htm

Car Wash
http://environment.about.com/od/greenlivingdesign/a/car_wash.htm
http://www.bts.gov/publications/state_transportation_profiles/state_transportation_
    statistics_2005/html/fast_facts.html
http://www.carcarecentral.com/admin/dhtml/inserts/image/image.asp?Pruuid=
    {6C3A8017-DA77-4F5F-98C5-007B5DD36F1A}

IN THE BACKYARD
Drip Irrigation
http://www.mwra.state.ma.us/04water/html/gardening.htm
http://www.nrdc.org/water/pollution/gsteps.asp
http://socialsciences.ucsc.edu/casfs/publications/cultivar/21.1.pdf

Existing Lawn Irrigation
http://www.siouxfalls.org/PublicWorks/Water/conservation/rebates.aspx
http://www.seminolecountyfl.gov/envsrvs/watercon/pdf/DownH2OBill.pdf
http://www.afcesa.af.mil/ces/cesc/water/AF%20Water%20Conservation%20Guidebook.pdf
http://www.lcra.org/water/landscape_irrigation.html#a1
http://www.epa.gov/water/you/chap1.html

Hoses
http://www.adirondackcouncil.org/energytips2.html
http://www.state.nj.us/drbc/dollars&sense.htm
http://worldwise.stores.yahoo.net/water.html
http://www.h2o4u.org/facts.html

Lawn Care
http://www.savingwater.org/docs/natlawncare.pdf

Pool
http://www.eastorange-nj.org/Departments/Water/Facts,%20Figures,%20Follies.htm
http://www.nspi.org/ProfessionalResources/Government+Relations/Facts+about+pool+
    water+usage.htm

Outdoor Lighting
http://www.energystar.gov/index.cfm?c=lighting.pr_lighting
See IDA Information Sheets http://www.darksky.org/ida/ida_2/info04.html and
    http://www.darksky.org/ida/ida_2/info26.html for additional energy-saving facts

Sprinklers
http://www.ci.concord.ca.us/living/recycle/env-water-use.htm
Worldwatch Institute, State of the World 2004 Special Focus: The Consumer Society,
    January 2004, ISBN: 0-393-32539-3

2

The Big Picture

http://www.cigarettelitter.org/index.asp?pagename=UN
http://www.p2pays.org/ref/06/05406.pdf
http://www.ehso.com/ehshome/batteries.php
http://www.summitglobal.com/acrobat_pdf/quick_water_supply_facts_jan_03.pdf

The Simple Steps

NAPKINS

http://www.green-networld.com/tips/paper.htm
http://www.wesleyan.edu/hermes/prev/oct98/HI.htm
http://www.foodservice.com/news/company_news_detail.cfm?id=9042&company_name
http://www.gp.com/csrr/environment/measures.html
http://www.kimberly-clark.com/aboutus
http://www.pegasuscom.com/tstart2.html
http://www.esbnyc.com/tourism/tourism_facts.cfm?CFID=46899

BATTERIES

http://www.informinc.org/fact_CWPbattery.php#bwps

TAP WATER

http://www.nrdc.org/water/drinking/bw/chap4.asp
http://www.emagazine.com/view/?1125
http://www.agiweb.org/gap/legis109/drought.html
http://costofwar.com/index-pre-school.html
http://container-recycling.org/mediafold/newsarticles/plastic/2006/5-WMW-DownDrain.htm

The Little Things

Albums

http://www.vinylinfo.org/environment/recycling.html

Books

http://www.ala.org/ala/alalibrary/libraryfactsheet/alalibraryfactsheet1.htm
http://www2.sims.berkeley.edu/research/projects/how-much-info-2003/print.htm
http://answers.google.com/answers/threadview?id=433693
http://www.alcoa.com/global/en/environment/pdf/one_million_trees.pdf

http://www.nytimes.com/2005/04/28/books/28groc.html?ex=1272340800&en=fdd8f284
b6beae7b&ei=5088&partner=rssnyt&emc=rss
http://www.tew.org/development/illiteracy.html
http://www.census.gov/Press-Release/www/releases/archives/miscellaneous/007871.html
http://www.coloradotrees.org/benefits.htm

Candy
http://www.mtholyoke.edu/offices/srm/env/recycle/paper.shtml

Compact Discs
http://www.usatoday.com/life/music/news/2004-04-18-worst-songs_x.htm
http://www.epa.gov/osw/students/finalposter.pdf

DVDs
http://www.npd.com/dynamic/releases/press_050602.html
http://www.naa.org/info/facts04/recycling.html

Gift Wrap
http://www.eco-artware.com/newsletter/newsletter_12_01.shtml
http://bg.catalogagemag.com/ar/marketing_tips_improve_site
http://www.marketresearch.com/map/prod/1170982.html

Invitations
http://www.rmi.org/sitepages/pid894.php

Magazines
http://www.magazine.org/Government_Action/Environment/

MP3 Players
http://playlistmag.com/features/2005/06/ewaste/index.php?lsrc=mwrss

Newspapers
http://www.ilacsd.org/recycle/trivia.html
http://web.mit.edu/facilities/environmental/recyc-facts.html
http://www.bcua.org/SolidWaste_Recycling.htm

Placeware
http://www.crafta.com/party-supply-party-decoration.html

Popcorn
http://www.popcorn.org/frames.cfm?main=/teachers/index.cfm&usernav=flash

Restaurants
http://www.p2pays.org/p2rx/nav.cfm?hub=448&subsec=3
http://www.ciwmb.ca.gov/foodwaste/FAQ.htm
http://www.organicconsumers.org/organic/compost110504.cfm

Soda
http://www.co.ba.md.us/Agencies/publicworks/recycling/recylfact.html

Televisions
http://quote.bloomberg.com/apps/news?pid=nifea&&sid=aROY9gOh42KM
http://www.nrdc.org/air/energy/energyeff/tv.pdf
http://www.worldwatch.org/node/1481
http://www.epa.gov/epaoswer/osw/students/finalposter.pdf
http://www.lake-online.com/nicc/nicc_news.html
http://www.nwf.org/nationalwildlife/article.cfm?issueID=77&articleID=1123
http://www.pristineplanet.com/newsletter/2005/04.asp

Tickets
http://www.boston.com/business/technology/articles/2003/08/24/e_mail_is_just_the_
    ticket?mode=PF
http://www.indiescene.net/archives/movie_marketing/market_research/

Videocameras
http://www.pcmag.com/article2/0,1895,1900006,00.asp
http://pages.ebay.com/services/sellingcenter/cameras/howmuch.html

3

The Big Picture

http://www.rff.org/Documents/RFF-DP-00-14.pdf
http://www.tia.org/pressmedia/domestic_a_to_z.html
http://www.hotelmotel.com/hotelmotel/article/articleDetail.jsp?id=170828
http://www.bts.gov/publications/1995_american_travel_survey/us_profile/entire.pdf
http://www.fathers.com/articles/articles.asp?id=613&cat=4
http://www.oceansatlas.org/servlet/CDSServlet?status=ND0xNzk0MCY2PWVuJjMzP
    SomMzc9a29z
http://www.natca.org/mediacenter/bythenumbers.msp
http://enn.com/biz.html?id=538

The Simple Steps

REUSE LINENS AND TOWELS
http://www.sbeap.org/ppi/publications/Lodging_Logic.pdf

PACK LIGHTLY
http://www.britishairways.com/flights/factfile/airfleet/docs/7474.shtml

GROUP TRAVEL
http://www.grist.org/news/counter/2001/08/29/skies

The Little Things

TRAVEL PLANNING
Adventure Travel
http://www.smartertravel.com/travel-advice/goodbye-mickey-hello-machu-picchu-family-
    adventure-travel-is-on-the-rise.html?id=1290008&page=2
http://www.bellaonline.com/ArticlesP/art10494.asp

Camera
http://www.kodak.com/eknec/PageQuerier.jhtml?pq-path=4242&pq-locale-=en_US
http://www.pmai.org/new_pma/Marketing_Research/Photo%20Industry%202004.pdf

Cruise
http://www.rff.org/Documents/RFF-DP-00-14.pdf
http://www.cruising.org/press/overview%202006/2.cfm
http://en.wikipedia.org/wiki/Freedom_of_the_Seas_(ship)

Eco-Tourism
http://www.ecotourism.org/index2.php?what-is-ecotourism

Guidebooks
http://www2.sims.berkeley.edu/research/projects/how-much-info/print.html
http://www.p2pays.org/ref/02/01031.pdf

Hotels
http://www.energystar.gov/index.cfm?c=hospitality.bus_hospitality
http://www.emediawire.com/releases/2005/10/emw295598.htm

Luggage Tags
http://www.ilea.org/lcas/Tellus.html

Maps
http://archive.greenpeace.org/toxics/reports/gopher-reports/papdam.txt
http://www.epa.gov/epaoswer/non-hw/muncpl/facts.htm

Ticketing
http://money.cnn.com/1998/06/23/travelcenter/biztravel_column/
http://www.iata.org/NR/rdonlyres/6E53D204-1CF2-4509-AC9D-01E2DAEDD845/0/
    IndustryTimesAugust.pdf
http://www.countryplace.com/cplace/Congress/Airline_Fairness.html

Time of Year
http://envirovaluation.org/
http://www.ustoa.com/pressroom/newsreleases/savings.html

Toiletries
http://wasteage.com/mag/waste_hdpe_bottles
http://www.stopwaste.org/home/index.asp?page=261
http://www.ucsusa.org/publications/greentips/304-lowimpact-travel-tips.html

LEAVING HOME
Appliances
http://www.post-gazette.com/pg/05128/500530.stm

Lights
http://www.topbulb.com/energystar
http://www.prnewswire.com/cgi-bin/stories.pl?ACCT=104&STORY=/www/story/07-03-2002/0001758477&EDATE=

Mail
http://www.usps.com/environment/_pdf/amail.pdf

Newspapers
http://www.naa.org/thesource/26.asp
http://www.bostonglobe.com/subscriber/info/faqs/faqcs.stm

Shades
http://www.eia.doe.gov/kids/energyfacts/saving/efficiency/savingenergy.html
http://www.curtainandbath.com/energy_saving_items.htm
http://www.bpa.gov/Energy/n/Energy_Tips/save_energy/heating.cfm

Thermostat
http://www.energytrust.org/residential/hes/es_heat_cool.html
http://www.eia.doe.gov/kids/energyfacts/saving/efficiency/savingenergy.html

GETTING THERE
Baggage
http://www.badcases.com/bad/restrictions/airlines.html

Check-In
http://thefuntimesguide.com
http://www.iata.org/NR/rdonlyres/6E53D204-1CF2-4509-AC9D-01E2DAEDD845/0/IndustryTimesAugust.pdf

Hybrid Car Service
http://www.msnbc.msn.com/id/8420904

Transportation
http://www.usatoday.com/travel/news/2006-06-23-airport-transfer-costs-x.htm?csp=34
http://www.delta.com/traveling_checkin/airport_information/airport_maps/atlanta_atl/index.jsp
http://www.bts.gov/press_releases/2006/bts020_06/html/bts020_06.html

AT THE HOTEL
Lights
http://www.ahla.com/products_info_center_lip.asp
http://www.lbl.gov/Science-Articles/Archive/EETD-lighting-demo.html
http://www.energystar.gov/ia/business/hospitality/factsheet_0804.pdf

Plugs/Adapters
http://www.solio.com/tradedownloads/solio_reseller/Solio%20Info.pdf
http://www.post-gazette.com/pg/05128/500530.stm

Washing Clothes
http://economicallysound.com/random_thoughts/index.html

SIGHTSEEING/GETTING AROUND
Car Rentals
http://www.fleet-central.com/arn/t_pop_pdf.cfm?action=stat&link=http://www.
    fleet-central.com/arn/stats/2005/U.S._Car_Rental_Market.pdf
http://www.runzheimer.com/web/publications/RRTM/rrtm-1999-10-v19-n6.pdf
http://www.fueleconomy.gov/feg/hybrid_sbs_cars.shtml
http://www.fueleconomy.gov/feg/findacar.htm

Locations
http://en.wikipedia.org/wiki/Colosseum
http://csdngo.igc.org/tourism/tourdial_coast.htm

Paths
http://www.audubon.org/market/no/ethic/index.html

Water Bottles
http://cbs2.com/topstories/topstories_story_019125500.html
http://en.wikipedia.org/wiki/Bottled_water
http://www.earth-policy.org/Updates/2006/Update51.htm

The Big Picture

http://www.epa.gov/epaoswer/hazwaste/recycle/ecycling/index.htm
http://www.boeing.com/defense-space/space/bss/sat101.html
http://www.technology.gov/speeches/p_BHW_050817.htm
http://www.washingtonpost.com/wp-dyn/content/article/2005/12/11/AR2005121100664
    .html
http://www.cleanairpartnership.org/cleanairguide/electronics/

The Simple Steps
CELL PHONE RECYCLING
http://www.worldwatch.org/node/1482
http://www.recyclemycellphone.org/faq.shtml#DEDUCTIBLE
http://www.eco-cell.org/cellwaste.asp

UNPLUG POWER
http://communityrelations.berkeley.edu/CalNeighbors/Spring2001/appliances.html
http://www.findarticles.com/p/articles/mi_m5072/is_47_24/ai_97616269

DOWNLOAD SOFTWARE
http://www.space.com/scienceastronomy/101_earth_facts_030722-4.html
http://www.conservation.org/xp/CIWEB/getinvolved/whatyoucando/athome.xml#6

http://infochangeindia.org/kids/trouble_05.jsp
http://en.wikipedia.org/wiki/Compact_disc

The Little Things

Answering Machines
http://www.eia.doe.gov/emeu/reps/enduse/er01_us_tab1.html
http://www.energystar.gov/index.cfm?fuseaction=find_a_product.showProductGroup&
    pgw_code=CL

Computers
http://www.energystar.gov/index.cfm?c=power_mgt.pr_power_management
http://www.svtc.org/cleancc/pubs/sayno.htm#clean.htm

Digital
http://en.wikipedia.org/wiki/Analog_television
http://www.nab.org/Newsroom/PressRel/Filings/OTAAtt81104.pdf
http://www.yesmagazine.org/article.asp?ID=1343

Discs
http://www.afterdawn.com/news/archive/5141.cfm
http://www.blu-ray.com/faq/#bluray

Headsets
http://www.ehso.com/ehshome/batteries.php

High-Speed Internet
http://www.eere.energy.gov/consumer/your_home/appliances/index.cfm/mytopic=10040
http://blogs.zdnet.com/ITFacts/?cat=2
http://www.humboldt.edu/~envecon/internet.html#envecon
http://www.ecomall.com/
http://firstmonday.org/issues/issue8_3/davison

Messaging
http://www.eia.doe.gov/emeu/reps/enduse/er01_us.html
http://www.lbl.gov/Science-Articles/Archive/data-center-energy-myth.html
http://searchmobilecomputing.techtarget.com/originalContent/0,289142,sid40_gci11933
    10,00.html
http://hpl.hp.com/techreports/2003/HPL-2003-167.pdf

Pagers
http://tech2.nytimes.com/mem/technology/techreview.html?res=980DE6DC1E3DF932A25
    757C0A9649C8B63

Personal Digital Assistants
http://www.kdheks.gov/waste/swupdate/SW_Update_0504.pdf
http://www.enviroliteracy.org/article.php/1119.html

Power Strips
http://www.lbl.gov/Science-Articles/Archive/leaking-watts.html

Power Usage
http://www.clickz.com/showPage.html?page=3559991
http://www.eu-energystar.org/en/en_022.htm
http://www.extrasys.com/whitepapers/pdfs/energy_study.pdf

The Big Picture

http://www.epa.state.il.us/p2/green-schools/green-schools-checklist.pdf
http://www.asbj.com/199901/0199coverstory.html
http://www.ase.org/content/article/detail/2977
http://www.energy.gov/news/1257.htm
http://www.vpirg.org/downloads/toxicschools.pdf

The Simple Steps

WASTE-FREE LUNCH
http://www.babybag.com/articles/htwt_av.htm
http://www.cdc.gov/growthcharts/
http://www.wastefreelunches.org/
http://www.informinc.org/getatlunch.php

WALK TO SCHOOL
http://www.nsc.org/ehc/mobile/mse_fs.htm
http://www.bts.gov/publications/transportation_statistics_annual_report/1999/chapter4/
     chap4.htm
http://www.ed.gov/about/offices/list/ous/international/usnei/us/edlite-primseced.html
http://walking.about.com/od/healthbenefits/a/livelonger1105.htm

PAPER
http://www.ciwmb.ca.gov/Schools/WasteReduce/Survey/default.asp
http://www.vermico.com/bookreview.html
http://www.officedepot.com/storeFront.do?Nr=100000&N=100000+300058

The Little Things

GETTING THERE
Bicycle
http://www.bicyclecommuter.com/AmericanGridlock.htm

Bus
http://www.grist.org/advice/possessions/2003/09/15/t
http://www.census.gov/Press-Release/www/releases/archives/
     facts_for_features_special_editions/005225.html
http://www.nlc.org/about_cities/cities_101/138.cfm

http://www.grist.org/news/counter/2001/08/29/skies/
http://www.publicpurpose.com/ut-scbpm2004.htm

Carpooling
http://www.epa.gov/rtirmd10/transportation/carpooling/emissions.htm

IN THE CLASSROOM
Blackboard Erasers
http://www.troydryerase.com/Chalk-Dust-Healthresearch.htm

Blackboards
http://www.nhlbi.nih.gov/health/public/lung/asthma/resolut.htm
http://www.epa.gov/iaq/schools/actions_to_improve_iaq.html

Chalk
http://www.nhlbi.nih.gov/health/public/lung/asthma/resolut.htm
http://www.epa.gov/iaq/schools/actions_to_improve_iaq.html

Crayons
http://dingo.care-mail.com/channels/!cgrwrit.pdf

Markers
http://dingo.care-mail.com/channels/!cgrwrit

Pens
http://dingo.care-mail.com/channels/!cgrwrit.pdf
http://www.p2ric.org/video/details_videoclip.cfm?chapter_id=115
http://www.epa.gov/superfund/students/clas_act/haz-ed/ff06.pdf

Pencils
http://www.care2.com/channels/solutions/home/66
http://dingo-care-mail.com/channels/!cgrwrit

Schoolbooks
http://www.publishers.org/industry/S1_04.pdf
http://money.cnn.com/2006/10/24/pf/college/college_costs/index.htm

Temperature
http://www.cefpi.org/epa_temperature.html

AT LUNCH
Food Donation
http://www.ciwmb.ca.gov/schools/WasteReduce/Food/Donation.htm

Food Types
http://www.wastefreelunches.org/
http://www.findarticles.com/p/articles/mi_m1355/is_19_99/ai_73890537
http://www.cehca.org/lunchbox_factsheet.pdf
http://mchb.hrsa.gov/chusa03/pages/population.htm

Gum
http://www.confectionerynews.com/news/ng.asp?n=65326&m=2CNE124&c=[emailcode]
http://factfinder.census.gov/servlet/STTable?_bm=y&-geo_id=01000US&-qr_name=
    ACS_2005_EST_G00_S0101&-ds_name=ACS_2005_EST_G00
http://www.checkout.ie/Feature.asp?ID=109
http://www.epa.gov/epaoswer/non-hw/muncpl/pubs/msw05rpt.pdf
http://www.parliament.uk/post/pn201.pdf
http://en.wikipedia.org/wiki/Metric_meterstick

Recycling
http://www.epa.gov/globalwarming/greenhouse/greenhouse18/school_kids.html

Vending Machines
http://www.usatoday.com/news/health/2004-05-11-vending-machines_x.htm
http://www.ncsl.org/programs/health/vending.htm
http://www.iom.edu/Object.File/Master/22/606/FINALfactsandfigures2.pdf
http://www.metro-region.org/article.cfm?articleid=5563

HOMEWORK
Library Books
http://www.nclis.gov/statsurv/summarystats.pdf
http://nces.ed.gov/pubs2005/2005356.pdf
http://en.wikipedia.org/wiki/Digital_library

SCHOOL SUPPLIES
Adhesive Notes
http://www.officedepot.com/textSearch.do?uniqueSearchFlag=true&Ntt=3m
http://www.rakemag.com/stories/section_detail.aspx?itemID=5383&catID=146&Select
    CatID=146

Binders
http://www.mead.com/webapp/wcs/stores/servlet/
    product3_10051_10006_125792_-1_false_10051

File Folders
http://www.easternct.edu/depts/amerst/MallsWorld.htm
http://www.csrwire.com/PressRelease.php?id=2867
http://www.dolphinblue.com/file-folders.html

Notebooks
http://www.eia.doe.gov/kids/energyfacts/saving/recycling/solidwaste/metals.html

Paper
http://www.epa.gov/epaoswer/non-hw/muncpl/landfill/land-air.pdf
http://www.epa.gov/epaoswer/non-hw/muncpl/pubs/msw05rpt.pdf
http://www.eurekarecycling.org/pdfs/Fact_Sheet_Fall_2006.pdf
http://www.who.int/mediacentre/factsheets/fs225/en/index.html

http://www.greenseal.org/resources/reports/CGR=P&W2.pdf
http://www.teachersdomain.org/3-5/sci/ess/earthsys/conserve/index.html

Paper Clips
http://www.associatedcontent.com/article/6047/the_many_uses_of_paper_clips.html
http://www.epa.gov/epaoswer/non-hw/muncpl/pubs/msw05rpt.pdf
http://www.treehugger.com/files/materials/recycled/

Plastic
http://www.epa.gov/msw/pubs/mswchar05.pdf
http://www.grist.org/advice/possessions/2003/09/15/

Plastic Rulers
http://christianteens.about.com/od/sermons/a/backtoschoolfaq.htm

Scissors
http://www.worldwise.com/recyclingsteel.html
http://www.grist.org/advice/possessions/2003/09/15/
http://www.epa.gov/epaoswer/non-hw/muncpl/msw99.htm

Tape Dispenser
http://www.epa.gov/msw/pubs/msw03rpt.pdf

Wastebaskets
http://www.eia.doe.gov/kids/energyfacts/saving/recycling/solidwaste/metals.html
http://pediatrics.about.com/cs/growthcharts2/f/avg_wt_male.htm

STUDENT HOUSING
Dorms
http://en.wikipedia.org/wiki/College_town
http://www.bls.gov/news.release/pdf/hsgec.pdf

Laundry
http://www.epa.gov/safewater/kids/water_trivia_facts.html
http://michaelbluejay.com/electricity/laundry.html
http://www.coinlaundry.org/resource_edu/business_over.html

The Big Picture

http://www.cleanair.org/Waste/wasteFacts.html
http://www.p2pays.org/ref/03/02366.pdf
http://www.fullcirclerecycling.com/faq.html
http://www.moea.state.mn.us/campaign/workplace/
http://www.wastecapwi.org/documents/officewaste.pdf
http://www.epa.gov/greenbuilding/pubs/gbstats.pdf

http://www.eia.doe.gov/kids/energyfacts/uses/commercial.html
http://www.lrc.rpi.edu/programs/
http://enn.com/biz.html?id=538
http://www.cqc.com/~ccswmd/trivia.htm

The Simple Steps

DOUBLE-SIDED COPIES
http://www.moea.state.mn.us/campaign/workplace/
http://www.bls.gov/opub/rtaw/pdf/table10.pdf
http://hypertextbook.com/facts/2001/JuliaSherlis.shtml
http://lyberty.com/encyc/articles/earth.html

CARPOOL
http://www.kiplingerforecasts.com/economic_outlook/tables/autos/autos_annual.htm
http://safety.fhwa.dot.gov/facts/index.htm

CERAMIC COFFEE MUGS
http://www.greenbiz.com/toolbox/howto_third.cfm?LinkAdvID=69658

The Little Things

GETTING THERE
Car
http://www.fueleconomy.gov/feg/maintain.shtml
http://www.idfa.org/facts/icmonth/page2.cfm

Public Transportation
http://www.publictransportation.org/reports/asp/pub_benefits.asp
http://www.bts.gov/publications/transportation_statistics_annual_report/2003/html/
    chapter_02/commuting_expenses_of_the_working_poor.html
http://www.bts.gov/press_releases/2003/bts020_03/html/bts020_03.html
http://www.portauthority.org/PAAC/News/NewsRoom/BenefitsofTransit/tabid/270/
    Default.aspx

Telecommute
http://www.telcoa.org/id33.htm
http://www.itsdocs.fhwa.dot.gov/JPODOCS/REPTS_TE/8083.pdf

Walk
http://www.scorecard.org/ranking/rank-states.tcl?how_many=100&drop_down_name=
    Air+releases
http://www.yvcog.org/ctr/ccframe.htm
http://walking.about.com/od/pedestrians/p/walktoworkday.htm
http://www.earth-policy.org/Books/Eco/EEch6_ss4.htm

IN THE BREAK ROOM
Coffeemaker
http://waterconservation.ifas.ufl.edu/trivia.htm

http://www.cia.gov/cia/publications/factbook/rankorder/2095rank.html
http://en.wikipedia.org/wiki/Coffee
http://www.ncausa.org/i4a/pages/index.cfm?pageID=32
http://www.africanwellfund.org/WWForum.html

Stirrers
http://www.nerdybooks.com/press/environment/environment_pr_041006.shtml

Sugars/Sweeteners
http://www.mindbranch.com/listing/product/R560-462.html
http://sugarbeet.ucdavis.edu/sugar_industry.html
http://agriculture.senate.gov/Hearings/06may10rooASAcharts.pdf
http://www.bayarearecycling.org/home/bayroc/Article-SaveMoney2002.doc

MEAL BREAKS
Cafeteria
http://www.georgiaconservancy.org/Education/TCSummer05.pdf
http://www.kab.org/programs.asp?id=532&rid=533
http://www.wasteonline.org.uk/resources/InformationSheets/WasteAtWork.htm
http://www.greenbiz.com/toolbox/howto_third.cfm?LinkAdvID=69658

Food Storage
http://greenearthofficesupply.stores.yahoo.net/biodcelbagfo.html
http://investor.conagrafoods.com/phoenix.zhtml?c=97518&p=irol-newsArticlemedia&ID=
    766497&highlight=

Litter
http://www.longwood.edu/CLEANVA/cigbuttimpacts.htm
http://www.falkirk.gov.uk/litterzone/strat/strat31.shtm

Lunch
http://web.ead.anl.gov/uranium/guide/facts/

Paper Napkins
http://www.hot-dog.org/facts/hd_vitalstats.htm
http://wesleyan.edu/hermes/prev/oct98/H1.htm
http://www.green-network.com/tips/paper.htm

Takeout
http://ladpw.org/epd/recycling/crm.cfm

IN THE SUPPLY ROOM
Copier
http://www.eia.doe.gov/basics/energybasics101.html
http://www.epa.gov/oaintrnt/content/energy/aware.htm#monitor
http://www.rechargermag.com/article.asp?id=199906060

Correction Fluid
http://www.jobbankusa.com/ohb/ohb151.html
http://en.wikipedia.org/wiki/Image:Wite-Out_123.PNG

Envelopes
http://yosemite.epa.gov/R10/HOMEPAGE.NSF/d7b03c22cbc0843588256464006a2ff4/
    a4bbc0525b85e52288256ff90072393b!OpenDocument
http://www.environmentaldefense.org/article.cfm?contentid=640

Fax Machines
http://www.environmentaldefense.org/article.cfm?contentid=39
http://www.comodogroup.com/products/fax/index.html

Labels
http://www.epa.gov/msw/paper.htm
http://www.greenseal.org/resources/reports/CGR_officesupplies.pdf
http://www.environmentaldefense.org/article.cfm?contentid=39

Packaging/Shipping
http://www.dnr.mo.gov/energy/eia-fossilfuel.htm
http://www.resourcesaver.org/file/toolmanager/O16F3108.pdf
http://www.environmentaldefense.org/article.cfm?contentid=640

Paper
http://www.anjr.com/resources/whyrecycle.html#Anchor-Why-65288
http://www.epa.gov/oaintrnt/content/energy/aware.htm#monitor

Paper Clips
http://www.sba.gov/gopher/Business-Development/Success-Series/Vol8/serving.txt
http://www.associatedcontent.com/article/6047/the_many_uses_of_paper_clips.html
http://www.epa.gov/epaoswer/non-hw/muncpl/pubs/msw05rpt.pdf
http://www.treehugger.com/files/materials/recycled

Pens
http://www.epenz.co.nz/why_epenz.htm
http://www.nytco.com/investors-presentations-20051207b.html
http://www.findarticles.com/p/articles/mi_m3374/is_n20_v13/ai_11538759
http://www.epa.gov/epaoswer/aging/home-off.pdf

Postage Meters
http://es.epa.gov/techinfo/specific/proj-sum.html
http://ribbs.usps.gov/files/fedreg/USPS2000/00-31359.TXT
http://www.stamps.com/innerspace/vs_postage_meters/

Printers
http://www.advancedbuildings.org/_frames/fr_t_motor_energy_eff_equip.htm
http://home.earthlink.net/~jimlux/artlight.htm
http://www.epa.gov/oaintrnt/content/energy/aware.htm#monitor

Recycle
http://www.state.co.us/oemc/programs/commercial/recycling/Commercial_Recycling_
     Report.pdf
http://www.ciwmb.ca.gov/LGLibrary/Innovations/MiniBins/

Rubber Bands
http://skyways.lib.ks.us/towns/Cawker/twine.html
http://www.npi.gov.au/database/substance-info/profiles/1.html
http://www.therubberband.info/history.php
http://pubs.acs.org/cen/coverstory/8115/8115rubber.html
http://www.dykemarubberband.com/docs/RubberbandHistory.pdf

Staples
http://tekgems.com/Products/tg-et-15659-msc-no-staples.htm
http://www.census.gov/industry/1/ma33b98.pdf
http://www.eia.doe.gov/emeu/efficiency/carbon_emissions/steel.html

AT YOUR DESK
Computers
http://pmdb.cadmusdev.com/powermanagement/quickCalc.html

Cooling
http://www.ceel.org/resrc/facts/hecac-fx.php3

E-Mail
http://www.email-policy.com/
http://www.sfgate.com/cgi-bin/article.cgi?f=/g/a/2005/07/11/wastingtime.TMP
http://enduse.lbl.gov/Projects/InfoTech.html
http://arstechnica.com/news.ar/post/2007215-8854.html

Heating
http://www.aceee.org/ogeece/ch1_index.htm
http://www.energyfinder.org/efficiency/measures/commercial/consumption.asp
http://www.ccohs.ca/oshanswers/phys_agents/thermal_comfort.html
http://www.eia.doe.gov/kids/energyfacts/uses/commercial.html
http://www.wisegeek.com/is-there-a-link-between-office-temperature-and-worker-
     productivity.htm

Lighting
http://www.habitablezone.com/space/messages/437841.html
http://www.blm.gov/nhp/pubs/brochures/EnergyBro.htm
http://www.eia.doe.gov/emeu/aer/pdf/pages/sec2_4.pdf
http://www.eia.doe.gov/kids/energyfacts/uses/commercial.html
http://www.eia.doe.gov/emeu/cbecs/cbecs2f.html
http://www.lrc.rpi.edu/programs/DELTA/pdf/DeltaSnap5.pdf

Virtual Meetings
http://eetd.lbl.gov/newsletter/cbs_nl/nl16/dcoffice.html

7

The Big Picture

http://retailindustry.about.com/
http://retailindustry.about.com/library/bl/q2/bl_jup052201.htm
http://nationalzoo.si.edu/Publications/GreenTeam/#Toothbrushes
http://www.epa.gov/msw/pubs/ex-sum05.pdf
http://www.worldbank.org/research/journals/wbro/obsaug95/waste.htm
http://www.answers.com/topic/human-weight
http://www.epa.gov/water/you/chap1.html
http://www.mcdonough.com/writings/new_geography.htm
http://www.stevetrash.com/booking/lessons/lesson6.htm
http://www.need.org/needpdf/infobook_activities/SecInfo/ConsS.pdf
http://www.epa.gov/industrialwaste/

The Simple Steps

PACKAGING

http://www.eia.doe.gov/kids/energyfacts/saving/recycling/solidwaste/sourcereduction.html
http://edis.ifas.ufl.edu/pdffiles/AE/AE22600.pdf
http://www.census.gov/Press-Release/www/releases/archives/miscellaneous/005262.html
http://wastec.isproductions.net/webmodules/webarticles/anmviewer.asp?a=459
http://en.wikipedia.org/wiki/Central_Park
http://www.amazon.com/gp/product/B0003298L2/ref=nosim/002-0775315-8511250?n=
    3370831
http://www.amazon.com/gp/product/B000BY8MZ0/qid=1156277260/sr=1-4/ref=sr_1_4/
    002-0775315-8511250?%5Fencoding=UTF8&n=3600731&s=gourmet-food&v=glance
http://www.enchantedlearning.com/history/us/monuments/whitehouse/

SHOPPING BAGS

http://www.findarticles.com/p/articles/mi_m1016/is_n1-2_v96/ai_8346997

BATHROOM TISSUE

http://www.drugstore.com/qxp89432_333181_sespider/seventh_generation/bath_tissue_
    double_rolls.htm

The Little Things

GROCERIES

Bread—Dinner

http://www.infra.kth.se/fms/pdf/food.i.ec.pdf
http://www.bts.gov/publications/national_transportation_statistics/2003/html/table_04_20
    .html
http://www.pbs.org/wnet/colonialhouse/print/p-teach_lesson1_answers.html

Bread—Sliced

http://www.nclnet.org/general/Package%20report/nclreport.htm
http://ask.yahoo.com/20061123.html

Bulk

http://books.google.com/books?id=JToDDMMQCfQC&dq=buying+in+bulk+percent+less+
    packaging&pg=PA275&ots=WElhNT565P&sig=8ePxdjmaVgydsgZPuByM-2_mqg&prev
    =http://www.google.com/search%3Fnum%3D30%26hl%3Den%26lr%3D%26q%3
    Dbuying%2Bin%2Bbulk%2Bpercent%2Bless%2Bpackaging&sa=X&oi=print&ct=
    result&cd=2
http://www.epa.gov/garbage/pubs/msw05rpt.pdf
http://www.johnmccrory.com/bags/v1/n13_5.html
http://www.epa.gov/garbage/pubs/wtsdmm.pdf
http://www.eere.energy.gov/cleancities/toolbox/pdfs/ggt.pdf
http://www.biodiesel.org/resources/users/stories/2004_0503_michigan_buses.pdf

Canned Goods

http://www.solidwaste.org/recdetin.htm
http://www.cancentral.com/standard.cfm#foodcan
http://www.epa.gov/msw/pubs/msw05rpt.pdf
http://www.energybulletin.net/14143.html
http://earthtrends.wri.org/pdf_library/data_tables/enel_2005.pdf
http://www.paris.org/Monuments/Eiffel/

Cheese

http://www.ers.usda.gov/data/FoodConsumption/spreadsheets/dymfg.xls#AmCheese!A1
http://www.p2pays.org/ref/08/07652.pdf
http://www.travelnotes.org/NorthAmerica/distances.htm
http://quickfacts.census.gov/qfd/states/55/5553000.html

Coffee

http://www.transfairusa.org/content/about/environmental.php
http://www.birdsandbeans.ca/richerEarth/SMBC.shtm
http://www.rainforest-alliance.org/cafe/english.html
http://www.thanksgivingcoffee.com/ceo/infopopups/shade_pk-zoosoc.html
http://www.publish.csiro.au/samples/1559633700.pdf
http://www.census.gov/compendia/statab/prices/prices.pdf
http://quickfacts.census.gov/qfd/states/53/5363000.html

Farmer's Market vs. Supermarket

http://www.worldwatch.org/node/827
http://www.sustainabletable.org/issues/energy/
http://www.randomhouse.com/catalog/display.pperl?isbn=9780767918343&view=
    excerpt&ref=emailcooking
http://www.worldwatch.org/node/1749

Fish—Farmed vs. Wild

http://www.nicholas.duke.edu/solutions/documents/pewreport.pdf

Fish—Fresh vs. Canned
http://www.agrifood-forum.net/publications/guide/f_chp2.pdf
http://hotdocs.usitc.gov/tata/hts/other/rel_doc/bill_reports/s--1739.pdf
http://www.bumblebee.com/pressroom_article4.jsp
http://www.tunafacts.com/industry/fast_facts.cfm
http://www.agry.purdue.edu/TURF/pubs/ay31.htm
http://sports.espn.go.com/outdoors/fishing/news/story?page=f_enc_YellowfinTuna

Fruit
http://baltimorechronicle.com/2006/071906climatecrisis.shtml
http://www.ers.usda.gov/data/fruitvegetablecosts/Fruits.xls
http://www.census.gov/prod/2005pubs/am0431gs1.pdf
http://www.census.gov/econ/census02/data/industry/E3114.HTM
http://www.ers.usda.gov/publications/agoutlook/aotables/2006/07Jul/aotab39.xls
http://www.eia.doe.gov/emeu/reps/enduse/er01_us_tab1.html

Meat
http://www.ers.usda.gov/Publications/foodreview/jan1997/jan97a.pdf
http://www.meatami.com/content/presscenter/factsheets_Infokits/FactSheetMeat
    ProductionandConsumption.pdf
http://earthsave.org/newsletters/water.htm
http://www.thegreenlife.org/eat_sustainable.html
http://www.niagarafallslive.com/Facts_about_Niagara_Falls.htm
http://www.amif.org/FactsandFigures/FactSheetMeatProductionandConsumption.pdf

Milk
http://www.umich.edu/~nppcpub/research/milkjuice.pdf
http://www.nclnet.org/general/Package%20report/nclreport.htm
http://www.ers.usda.gov/data/foodconsumption/FoodAvailQueriable.aspx#midForm
http://www.ers.usda.gov/publications/ah697/ah697.pdf
http://www.eia.doe.gov/emeu/reps/enduse/er01_us_tab1.html

Organic
http://foodnews.org/highpest.php?prod=PFR20N01&
http://www.worldwatch.org/node/1761
http://www.ewg.org/reports/sludgememo/sludge.html

Paper Bags
http://www.thegreenguide.org/article/home/paper
http://www.epa.gov/region1/communities/shopbags.html
http://adminserv.depaul.edu/iprint/HTML/impact.html
http://www.nycvisit.com/content/index.cfm?pagePkey=57

Paper Towels
http://www.keysan.com/ksupa31.htm
http://wastec.isproductions.net/webmodules/webarticles/anmviewer.asp?a=463&z=44

Plastic Bags

http://www.nrdc.org/onearth/03sum/bag.asp
http://www.epa.gov/region1/communities/shopbags.html
http://www.eia.doe.gov/emeu/reps/enduse/er01_us_tab1.html
http://www.eia.doe.gov/kids/energyfacts/science/energy_calculator.html

Poultry

http://www.ers.usda.gov/Publications/foodreview/jan1997/jan97a.pdf
http://www.meatami.com/content/presscenter/factsheets_Infokits/FactSheetMeat
    ProductionandConsumption.pdf
http://cires.colorado.edu/~maurerj/vegetarian.htm
http://www.pe.com/localnews/politics/stories/PE_News_Local_D_lawns13.20595c2.html
http://www.50states.com/californ.htm

Soy

http://www.sierraclub.org/sustainable_consumption/toolkit/choosing.pdf

Trash Bags

http://www.naturallyhome.com/prod/12LT15.htm
http://www.ag.ndsu.edu/pubs/ageng/structu/ae1015.htm

Vegetables

http://www.census.gov/prod/2005pubs/am0431gs1.pdf
http://www.census.gov/econ/census02/data/industry/E3114.HTM
http://www.ers.usda.gov/publications/agoutlook/aotables/2006/07Jul/aotab39.xls
http://www.ers.usda.gov/data/fruitvegetablecosts/Vegetables.xls
http://www.ext.colostate.edu/PUBS/foodnut/08704.html
http://www.oag.state.ny.us/consumer/tips/energy_conservation.html

CLOTHING
Dyes

http://www.p2pays.org/ref/01/00506.pdf
http://www.coopamerica.org/pubs/realmoney/articles/backtoschoolclothes.cfm
http://ga.water.usgs.gov/edu/earthrain.html

Fabric

http://toxics.usgs.gov/regional/cotton.html
http://ipm.ncsu.edu/Production_Guides/Cotton/chptr1.pdf
http://usda.mannlib.cornell.edu/usda/ers/CWS//2000s/2006/CWS-05-15-2006.pdf
http://www.cotton.org/pubs/cottoncounts/what-can-you-make.cfm
http://www.p2pays.org/ref/33/32130.pdf

Fur

http://www.treehugger.com/files/2006/02/what_should_my.php
http://a257.g.akamaitech.net/7/257/2422/01jan20051800/edocket.access.gpo.gov/2005/
    pdf/E5-7531.pdf
http://infurmation.com/facts.php

Secondhand Clothing
http://www.essexcc.gov.uk/vip8/ecc/ECCWebsite/content/binaries/documents/waste/
    Chapter_6_Textiles.pdf?channelOid=null
http://hollywood.areaconnect.com/statistics.htm
http://www.bts.gov/publications/national_transportation_statistics/2003/html/table_04_20
    .html
http://www.laalmanac.com/transport/tr53.htm
http://www.eia.doe.gov/kids/energyfacts/science/energy_calculator.html

Shoes
http://www.g-forse.com/archive/news492_e.html
http://findarticles.com/p/articles/mi_m1594/is_n1_v8/ai_19192515
https://www.apparelandfootwear.org/UserFiles/File/Statistics/ShoeStats2005.pdf
http://www.eia.doe.gov/emeu/reps/enduse/er01_us_tab1.html

HEALTH
Homeopathic vs. Manufactured Pharmaceuticals
http://www.guna.it/eng/ricerca/prefazione.htm
http://www.epa.gov/compliance/resources/publications/assistance/sectors/notebooks/
    pharma.pdf
http://www.productstewardship.net/productsPharmaceuticals.html
http://www.nature.com/embor/journal/v5/n12/full/7400307.html

Prescription Medication
http://www.ehponline.org/members/2003/5948/5948.pdf
http://www.nature.com/embor/journal/v5/n12/full/7400307.html
http://www.phrma.org/files/2006%20Industry%20Profile.pdf
http://www.worstpills.org/public/page.cfm?op_id=3#
http://www.productstewardship.net/productsPharmaceuticals.html

Vitamins
http://www.hsph.harvard.edu/cancer/risk/multivitamins/basics/multivitamin_bet.htm
http://www.fda.gov/ola/2001/dietary.html
http://www.ozonelayer.noaa.gov/science/basics.htm

PETS
Collars/Leashes
http://www.all-you-want-to-know-about-dogs.com/Dog-leashes-collars.cfm
http://www.greenhome.com/products/pets/pet_accessories/105100/
http://www.shopping.com/xDN-Pets--dogs-9689_amazon-collars_and_leashes-standard_
    leashes-material_cotton
http://www.greenseal.org/resources/reports/CGR_carpet.pdf
http://www.trailcenter.org/newsletter/2000/spring2000/spring2000-06.htm
http://www.p2pays.org/ref/13/12044.pdf
http://yosemite.epa.gov/oar/globalwarming.nsf/content/ResourceCenterPublications
    GHGEmissionsUSEmissionsInventory2006Tables.html/$File/Table%20ES-3.csv

Fish Tanks

http://www.associatedcontent.com/article/11823/how_to_clean_your_fish_tank.html?
   page=2
http://www.bwsc.org/Community/conservation/tips.htm
http://www.nhmag.com/master.html?http://www.nhmag.com/0304/0304_feature.html
http://www.globalgreen.org/programs/water/index.html

Pet Beds

http://www.epa.gov/epaoswer/non-hw/recycle/recmeas/docs/guide_b.pdf
http://www.hsus.org/pets/issues_affecting_our_pets/pet_overpopulation_and_
   ownership_statistics/us_pet_ownership_statistics.html
http://www.greenhome.com/products/pets/pet_accessories/103481/
http://www.worldwise.com/poandsmbrshn.html

Pet Food

http://abcnews.go.com/GMA/story?id=1905511&page=4
http://www.vegansociety.com/html/environment/energy/
http://www.onlineconversion.com/energy.htm
http://www.avma.org/membshp/marketstats/sourcebook.asp

Pet Toys

http://www.appma.org/press_releasedetail.asp?v=ALL&id=84
http://www.hsus.org/pets/issues_affecting_our_pets/pet_overpopulation_and_
   ownership_statistics/us_pet_ownership_statistics.html
http://www.eia.doe.gov/emeu/reps/enduse/er01_us_tab1.html
http://quickfacts.census.gov/qfd/index.html
http://www1.shopping.com/xDN-Pets--dogs-pet_toys-pt_material_plastic~PG-1?NPP=90#stt
http://www.dogtoys.com/flyinfristoy.html
http://www.greendogonline.com/green_dog_gazette_11_04.pdf

Pet Treats

http://www.appma.org/press_releasedetail.asp?v=ALL&id=84
http://www.findarticles.com/p/articles/mi_m0EIN/is_2005_April_27/ai_n13656042
http://www.hsus.org/pets/issues_affecting_our_pets/pet_overpopulation_and_ownership_
   statistics/us_pet_ownership_statistics.html
http://www.shopping.com/xDN-pets--%3Efood_and_treats%5Eor-dogs-pt_food_and_
   treats_type_treats-price_range_0_10

LAWN AND GARDEN
Fertilizers

http://www.fcgov.com/recycling/basics.php
http://www.greenviewfertilizer.com/online/fertilizer_facts.jsp
http://www.energybulletin.net/281.html
http://www.american-lawns.com/lawns/lawn_benefits.html
http://www.amtrak.com/servlet/ContentServer?pagename=Amtrak/am2Copy/Title_
   Image_Copy_Page&c=am2Copy&cid=1093554056875&ssid=565

Floral Arrangements
http://www.ecobusinesslinks.com/organic_flowers.htm
http://www.nrdc.org/thisgreenlife/pdf/0503.pdf
http://www.theecologist.org/archive_detail.asp?content_id=230
http://www.zmag.org/content/Colombia/cox_flowers.cfm
http://www.johnson.cornell.edu/internationaleducation/politics/cases/Environment%20
    and%20Labor%20in%20the%20Colombian%20Flower%20Industry.doc
http://www.bestfrog.com/dash/index.php?sid=H&mid=3
http://www.funtrivia.com/askft/Question43743.html

Flowers
http://www.epa.gov/owow/NPS/dosdont.htm
http://www.usagreen.org/waterConservation.html
http://quickfacts.census.gov/qfd/states/06000.html
http://www.nwf.org/nationalwildlife/article.cfm?articleId=928&issueId=68

Outdoor Furniture
http://www.marmaxproducts.co.uk/recycling.asp
http://www.masonrymagazine.com/3-04/outdoor.html
http://plasticlumberyard.com/FURNITURE/garden48inchbenchGB48.htm

Sprinklers
http://www.worldwise.com/water2.html
http://www.seminolecountyfl.gov/envsrvs/watercon/pdf/DownH2OBill.pdf

KIDS
Baby Body Wash
http://www.checnet.org/healthehouse/education/articles-detail.asp?Main_ID=628
http://www.cdc.gov/nchs/fastats/births.htm
http://www.amazon.com/Primo-Eurobath-Color-Mint-Green/dp/B00078RVT8

Baby Food
http://www.ewg.org/reports/Baby_food/baby4.html
http://www.checnet.org/healthehouse/education/quicklist-detail.asp?Main_ID=241
http://www.nclnet.org/general/Package%20report/nclreport.htm
http://www.cspinet.org/reports/cheat1.html
http://www.planepage.com/Factsheets/index.php?TPPF_SearchString=2&TPPF_Search
    Category=ID&TPPF_Extended=yes

Baby Lotion
http://www.checnet.org/healthehouse/education/articles-detail.asp?Main_ID=628
http://www.plasticsresource.com/s_plasticsresource/rpd_product.asp?CID=86&DID=539&/
    Packaging/Skin+and+Personal+Care/952
http://www.cpcpkg.com/magazine/02_09_ondisplaytubes.php
http://www.accessexcellence.org/AE/AEPC/WWC/1991/waste.html
http://www.cdc.gov/nchs/fastats/births.htm

Baby Shampoo

http://www.amazon.com/s/ref=nb_ss_ba/103-8709322-4306242?url=searchalias%
    3Dbaby-products&field-keywords=shampoo
http://www.cdc.gov/nchs/fastats/births.htm

Baby Wipes

http://www.seventhgeneration.com/our_products/baby/baby_wipes.html
http://www.amazon.com/s/ref=sr_pg_2/103-8709322-4306242?ie=UTF8&
    keywords=wipes&rh=n%3A165797011%2Ck%3Awipes%2Cp%5F3%3A%240-
    %2424&page=2
http://www.ecologycenter.org/ptf/report1996/report1996_01.html
http://www.cdc.gov/nchs/fastats/births.htm
http://www.mid.org/services/save/hm-appl-cost-2005.htm

Batteries

http://www.checnet.org/healthehouse/education/articles-detail.asp?Main_ID=144
http://www.amazon.com/Maxell-Alkaline-Batteries-Value-Pack/dp/B0000Y3KS0/sr=
    8-1/qid=1158170511/ref=pd_bbs_1/103-8709322-4306242?ie=UTF8&s=
    electronics
http://www.census.gov/population/socdemo/hh-fam/p20-537/2000/tabC1.xls
http://www.corrosion-doctors.org/Batteries/cost.htm
http://www.avt.uk.com/page3.html
http://geography.about.com/library/faq/blqzcircumference.htm

Cloth vs. Disposable Diapers

http://www.mothering.com/articles/new_baby/diapers/politics.html
http://www.ecocycle.org/pdfs/Eco-facts_2004.pdf

Cotton Swabs

http://www.setterstix.com/cotton_swabs.php
http://www.madehow.com/Volume-4/Cotton-Swab.html
http://www.ecplaza.net/ecmarket/list.asp?cmd=search&keywords=cotton+swab&min_
    regdate=&cat=&country=CN&x=25&y=4
http://matse1.mse.uiuc.edu/polymers/h.html
http://www.ecologycenter.org/ptf/report1996/report1996_01.html
http://www.eia.doe.gov/emeu/reps/enduse/er01_us_tab1.html

Laundry Soap

http://www.shaklee.com/00128.html
http://www.eia.doe.gov/kids/energyfacts/science/energy_calculator.html

Strollers

http://www.shopping.com/xPP-Strollers—carriage
http://www.cdc.gov/nchs/fastats/births.htm
http://www.cpws.com/Appliance%20Use%20Chart.pdf

Toy Manufacturers
http://www.globalissues.org/TradeRelated/Consumption/Children.asp
http://www.checnet.org/healthehouse/education/quicklist-detail.asp?Main_ID=383
http://www.ban.org/ban_news/asias_wind.html

Toys
http://www.checnet.org/healthehouse/education/quicklist-detail.asp?Main_ID=645
http://www.environmentcalifornia.org/uploads/B0/av/B0avehMELtJWs0ZmzXiK4w/
    Shoppers_Guide.pdf
http://uspirg.org/reports/shoppingguidetoxics.pdf
http://www.shopping.com/xDN-baby_care—teethers__teething_rings
http://www.ecologycenter.org/ptf/report1996/report1996_01.html
http://www.cdc.gov/nchs/fastats/births.htm
http://www.energystar.gov/ia/partners/prod_development/revisions/downloads/tv_vcr/
    Ecos_Presentation.pdf

Toy Packaging
http://www.checnet.org/healthehouse/education/quicklist-detail.asp?Main_ID=383
http://www.hopkinsmn.com/community/environment/holidaywastereductiontips.html
http://www.globalissues.org/TradeRelated/Consumption/Children.asp
http://www.fne.asso.fr/preventiondechets/docs/etude_pakaging_wasteAutrichien.pdf
http://www.motherjones.com/news/outfront/1996/09/homeplanet.html
http://www.businessworld.in/oct1104/invogue01.asp
http://www.eplanettoys.com/store/comersus_index.asp

Toys—Plastic
http://www.checnet.org/healthehouse/education/quicklist-detail.asp?Main_ID=383
http://www.checnet.org/healthehouse/education/articles-detail.asp?Main_ID=136
http://www.greenpeace.org/raw/content/usa/press/reports/review-of-the-availability-of.pdf
http://uspirg.org/reports/troubleintoyland2005.pdf
http://www.youthnoise.com/page.php?page_id=470
http://www.globalissues.org/TradeRelated/Consumption/Children.asp
http://www.mid.org/services/save/hm-appl-cost-2005.htm
http://www.ecologycenter.org/ptf/report1996/report1996_01.html
http://www.census.gov/population/socdemo/hh-fam/p20-537/2000/tabC1.xls
http://amazon.com/s/ref=br_ss_hs/103-8709322-4306242?platform=gurupa&url=
    index%3Dtoys-and-games&keywords=plastic

Toys—Wood
http://www.checnet.org/healthehouse/education/quicklist-detail.asp?Main_ID=383
http://www.checnet.org/healthehouse/education/articles-detail.asp?Main_ID=136
http://www.greenpeace.org/raw/content/usa/press/reports/review-of-the-availability-of.pdf
http://www.census.gov/population/socdemo/hh-fam/p20-537/2000/tabC1.xls

HOLIDAYS
Candles
http://www.articlesbase.com/environment-articles/soy-vs-paraffin-candles--the-great-
    debate-39919.html

http://www.healthycandles.org/beeswax_candles.php
http://www.eia.doe.gov/pub/oil_gas/petroleum/analysis_publications/petroleum_
    profile_1999/profile99v8.pdf
http://www.eia.doe.gov/kids/energyfacts/science/energy_calculator.html
http://www.mid.org/services/save/hm-appl-cost-2006.htm
http://www.usnews.com/usnews/news/articles/051205/5datebook.htm

Christmas Trees
http://www.thegreenguide.com/doc.mhtml?i=61&s=christmastree
http://www.greenstarinc.org/enews/enewsv6n12.php
http://magazine.audubon.org/audubonathome/audubonathome0511.html
http://www.ctcns.com/fake-real.pdf
http://www.thegreenguide.com/doc.mhtml?i=ask&s=christmastree
http://www.audubon.org/bird/at_home/Holiday_Greening/treetrim.html
http://www.valentine.gr/enviroment-chrtees_en.htm

Decorations
http://www.audubon.org/bird/at_home/Holiday_Greening/treetrim:html
http://www.sfenvironment.com/facts/holidaytips/index.htm
http://frugalliving.about.com/gi/dynamic/offsite.htm?zi=1/XJ&sdn=frugalliving&zu=http%
    3A%2F%2Fwww.unitymarketingonline.com%2Freports2%2Fchristmas%2Fpr1.html
http://www.mid.org/services/save/hm-appl-cost-2005.htm

Gift Giving
http://www.audubon.org/bird/at_home/Holiday_Greening/gift_giving.html
http://news.nationalgeographic.com/news/2001/12/1221_holidaywasteline.html

Greeting Cards
http://www.thegreenguide.com/doc.mhtml?i=93&s=greetingcards
http://www.audubon.org/bird/at_home/Holiday_Greening/conserving.html
http://www.eia.doe.gov/kids/energyfacts/saving/recycling/solidwaste/paperandglass.html
http://www.mid.org/services/save/hm-appl-cost-2005.htm

Holiday Lights
http://www.eia.doe.gov/kids/energyfacts/science/energy_calculator.html
http://www.pge.com/news/news_releases/q4_2004/041124.html

Ribbons and Bows
http://geography.about.com/library/faq/blqzcircumference.htm
http://www.audubon.org/bird/at_home/Holiday_Greening/conserving.html

Wrapping Paper
http://www.audubon.org/bird/at_home/Holiday_Greening/party_planning.html
http://www.nrdc.org/reference/picks/pick0512.asp
http://quickfacts.census.gov/qfd/states/36/3651003.html

WINE AND BEER
Beverage Packaging
http://www.ratebeer.com/Story.asp?StoryID=385
http://www.consrv.ca.gov/index/news/2001%20News%20Releases/NR2001-51%20--
%20Recycling%20Commentary,%20Darryl%20Young.htm
http://www.aluminum.org/Template.cfm?Section=Home&template=/ContentManagement/
ContentDisplay.cfm&ContentID=5511
http://www.nbwa.org/Nbwa/faq
http://www.eia.doe.gov/kids/energyfacts/science/energy_calculator.html
http://www.bts.gov/publications/national_transportation_statistics/2003/html/
table_04_20.html

Domestic vs. Imported
http://www.acfonline.org.au/news.asp?news_id=491
http://www.infoplease.com/ipa/A0759496.html
http://www.thegreenguide.com/reports/product.mhtml?id=37
http://www.alcoholstats.com/mm/docs/2827.pdf
http://www.startribune.com/1229/story/893898.html

Organic Wine
http://www.wineinstitute.org/industry/statistics/2006/wine_sales.php
http://www.ers.usda.gov/data/FoodConsumption/FoodAvailQueriable.aspx#midForm
http://migration.ucdavis.edu/rmn/more.php?id=1116_0_5_0
http://www.birminghamweekly.com/archived/pages/20041223_food.php
http://www.teammahaska.org/php/archives.php
http://www.pesticideinfo.org/DS.jsp?sk=29143
http://coststudies.ucdavis.edu/uploads/cost_return_articles/grapewineim2005.pdf

MOTOR VEHICLES
Biodiesel
http://www.thegreenguide.com/doc.mhtml?i=91&s=biodiesel
http://www.sciam.com/article.cfm?chanID=sa003&articleID=BAF4F1A5938B8D520B328C
13B51CCF11
http://forums.tdiclub.com/showthread.php?t=149042
http://www.schoolbusinfo.org/intro.htm
http://www.azstarnet.com/sn/related/72010.php

Fuel
http://en.wikipedia.org/wiki/Octane_rating
http://www.p2pays.org/ref/13/12128.pdf

Hybrid
http://en.wikipedia.org/wiki/SULEV
http://www.suv.org/economic.html
http://www.nwma.org/pdf/miiMineralsBaby2004.pdf

http://www.sciam.com/article.cfm?chanID=sa003&articleID=BAF4F1A5938B8D520B328C13B51CCF11
http://auto.howstuffworks.com/question417.htm

Oil

http://www.epa.gov/cpg/pdf/vehicle.pdf
http://www.dtsc.ca.gov/PollutionPrevention/upload/re-refined-oil-fact-sheet.pdf
http://www.epa.gov/epaoswer/hazwaste/usedoil/usedoil.htm
http://www.commuter-register.org/crfuel.html
http://en.wikipedia.org/wiki/Energy_policy_of_the_United_States

PZEV

http://en.wikipedia.org/wiki/PZEV
http://www.grist.org/advice/possessions/2003/12/16/

Services

http://evolimo.com/cars.html
http://www.ozocar.com/
http://www.ag.state.mn.us/CONSUMER/ylr/ylr_06_Sept.htm
http://www.schallerconsult.com/taxi/taxifb.pdf
http://www.hybridcars.com/hybrid-taxicabs.html

Tires

http://www.epa.gov/cpg/pdf/vehicle.pdf
http://www.healthgoods.com/education/Environment_Information/Solid_Waste/tires.htm
http://www.p2pays.org/ref/04/03774.pdf

Used Vehicles

http://www.greencars.com
http://www.recycle-steel.org/PDFs/brochures/auto.pdf
http://www.nwma.org/pdf/miiMineralsBaby2004.pdf
http://goldengatebridge.org/research/factsGGBDesign.php

LUXURY ITEMS
Boats

http://www.ucsusa.org/publications/greentips/704-good-clean-boating-fun.html
http://www.ehponline.org/members/2003/111-4/focus.html

China

http://claymin.geoscienceworld.org/cgi/reprint/39/1/1
http://environment.about.com/od/greenlivingdesign/a/dishwashers.htm
http://www.topweddinglinks.com/wedding_statistics.html
http://home.howstuffworks.com/lenox1.htm
http://www.amazon.com/Mikasa-Platinum-5-Piece-Setting-Service/dp/B00004YNZY
http://www.mpw.org/exceldocs/energyuse.XLS

Crystal
http://www.lenntech.com/aquatic/metals-lead.htm
http://www.p2pays.org/ref/06/05458.pdf
http://www.mcswmd.org/Miscellaneous/Trivia.html
http://www.dld123.com/q&a/index.php?category=Food
http://meridianeng.com/lead.html

Diamonds
http://www.debeersgroup.com/NR/rdonlyres/847C1B2E-F3D2-461A-8BE3-E797DBF
    602DE/253/AR2001EnviroSustainability.pdf

Gold Jewelry
http://www.worldwatch.org/node/1491
http://www.sierraclub.org/trade/faces/pacific_rim.asp

Motorcycles
http://www.nrdc.org/bushrecord/2003_12.asp
http://www.epa.gov/oms/regs/nonroad/2002/f02039.pdf
http://www.bts.gov/publications/national_transportation_statistics/excel/table_04_11.xls
http://www.ersys.com/usa/32/3240000/distance.htm

Motor Homes
http://rvtravel.com/rvforum/viewtopic.php?p=3236&
http://www.familyrv.com/faq/faq-Motorhomes_vs_trailers.shtml
http://www.rversonline.org/MHvFW.html

Silver
http://findarticles.com/p/articles/mi_m1318/is_7_54/ai_63127427/pg_1
http://www.epa.gov/ttn/atw/urban/18catmem.pdf
http://www.eere.energy.gov/industry/steel/pdfs/theoretical_minimum_energies.pdf
http://www.eere.energy.gov/industry/mining/pdfs/gold-silver.pdf
http://www.deq.state.ok.us/LPDnew/education/recyclingfact.pdf
http://homepages.waymark.net/mikefirth/techspec.htm#MELTINGP
http://www.topweddinglinks.com/wedding_statistics.html
http://www.mpw.org/exceldocs/energyuse.XLS

ELECTRONICS
Computers
http://www.energystar.gov/index.cfm?fuseaction=find_a_product.showProductGroup&pgw
    _code=CO

DVD Players
http://www.energystar.gov/ia/business/bulk_purchasing/bpsavings_calc/Calc_DVD_
    Players.xls
http://www.dvdinformation.com/News/press/010903.htm
http://www.rtoonline.com/Content/Article/Jul04/100MillionDVDPlayers071604.asp

http://www.dvdforum.org/press-nd8-30-05.htm
http://www.eia.doe.gov/neic/experts/expertanswers.html

Fax Machines
http://eetd.lbl.gov/EA/Reports/46212/
http://www.columbia.edu/cu/environment/excel-files/Columbia_Computer_Energy_
    Usage_Calculator.xls
http://www.businessknowhow.com/homeoffice/whoworks.htm
http://h10010.www1.hp.com/wwpc/pscmisc/vac/us/product_pdfs/1834568.pdf
http://www2.sims.berkeley.edu/research/projects/how-much-info/print.html

Laptops vs. Desktops
http://www.mid.org/services/save/hm-appl-cost-2006.htm
http://www.svep.org/2003_index/2003%20SVEP%20Index.pdf
http://quickfacts.census.gov/qfd/states/06/06085.html

Mobile Phones
http://www.epa.gov/epaoswer/education/pdfs/life-cell.pdf
http://www.epa.gov/epaoswer/hazwaste/recycle/ecycling/index.htm

Personal Digital Assistants
http://www.informinc.org/fact_CWPbattery.php
http://www.springerlink.com/content/y13n30h3581b941j/fulltext.pdf

Phones
http://grist.org/advice/ask/2006/01/30/phones/index.html
http://eetd.lbl.gov/EA/Reports/46212/
http://www.oregonlive.com/cgi-bin/prxy/accessor/nph-repository-cache.cgi/base/
    pdf_captions/1164421507109810.pdf

Refurbished Computers
http://www.deq.state.ok.us/pubs/lpd/SecretLife_Computer.pdf
http://www.csc.calpoly.edu/~jdalbey/Public/secretlife.html
http://pubs.usgs.gov/fs/fs060-01/fs060-01.pdf
http://www.sahra.arizona.edu/programs/water_cons/home/pool_main.htm
http://www.census.gov/prod/2005pubs/p23-208.pdf

Stereos
http://www.npr.org/templates/story/story.php?storyId=5375728

Televisions
http://reviews.cnet.com/4520-6475_7-6400401-3.html
http://www.nrdc.org/air/energy/energyeff/tv.pdf

Video Game Consoles
http://reviews.cnet.com/Microsoft_Xbox_360/4505-6464_7-31355096.html
http://forum.pcvsconsole.com/viewthread.php?tid=11067

8

The Big Picture

http://www.fitcommerce.com/Blueprint/Module/Desktop/Announcements/
    ViewAnnouncement.aspx?ItemID=918&mid=112&tabId=87&tabIndex=0
http://www.msnbc.msn.com/id/3076635/
http://www.jrussellshealth.com/chemsensperf.html
http://www.ewg.org/issues/siteindex/issues.php?issueid=5026
http://www.stylecareer.com/tanningsalon_owner.shtml
http://www.findarticles.com/p/articles/mi_m0KFY/is_12_20/ai_98488428
http://nationalzoo.si.edu/Publications/GreenTeam/#Toothbrushes
http://www.pp.wmich.edu/rs/newsletters/fall06.pdf
http://www.bcua.org/SolidWaste_Recycling.htm

The Simple Steps

WATER BOTTLES
http://www.ciwmb.ca.gov/lglibrary/DSG/lRecycl.htm
http://www.bcua.org/SolidWaste_Recycling.htm
http://www.fitcommerce.com/Blueprint/Module/Desktop/Announcements/
    ViewAnnouncement.aspx?ItemID=918&mid=112&tabId=87&tabIndex=0

RAZORS
http://www.grist.org/advice/ask/2005/06/06/umbra-shaving/
http://www.ecologycenter.org/ptf/report1996/report1996_01.html
http://www.mid.org/services/save/hm-appl-cost-2006.htm
http://www.bts.gov/publications/national_transportation_statistics/2003/html/table_04_20.
    html
http://www.webflyer.com/travel/milemarker/getmileage.php?city=SAN&city=kona+hi

WALKING/JOGGING
http://www.chicagosolarpartnership.org/clientuploads/pdf/PiggyGuide2004.pdf?
    PHPSESSID=f90b15129b1245266a47ea07074cc605
http://www.walkaboutmag.com/17heller.html
http://www.tv.com/the-amazing-race/4-continents-24-cities-40000-miles/episode/
    395190/summary.html

The Little Things

AT THE GYM
Equipment
http://www.chicagosolarpartnership.org/clientuploads/pdf/PiggyGuide2004.pdf?
    PHPSESSID=f90b15129b1245266a47ea07074cc605
http://www.eia.doe.gov/kids/energyfacts/science/energy_calculator.html
http://www.nutristrategy.com/activitylist3.htm

Sauna/Steamroom
http://www.sdge.com/forms/energycosts.pdf

http://www.greatsaunas.com/information/us051.cfm
http://www.eia.doe.gov/emeu/reps/enduse/er01_us_tab1.html

Showering
http://www.ohiodnr.com/water/pubs/pdfs/fctsht01.pdf
http://www.meredithpools.com/estimate_gallons.htm

Towels
http://michaelbluejay.com/electricity/laundry.html
http://www.fitcommerce.com/Blueprint/Module/Desktop/Announcements/
    ViewAnnouncement.aspx?ItemID=918&mid=112&tabId=87&tabIndex=0
http://shopping.yahoo.com/s:Washers:2060-Washer%20Capacity=Large%
    20Capacity%20Washers
http://health.howstuffworks.com/how-to-live-with-allergies1.htm
http://www.dailymail.co.uk/pages/live/articles/health/healthmain.html?in_article_
    id=339623&in_page_id=1774&in_a_source

OUTDOOR EXERCISE
Biking
http://www.hc-sc.gc.ca/ewh-semt/pubs/air/active-transport-actif_e.html
http://www.sparetheair.com/publications/DirtyAirBooklet2004.pdf
http://www.grist.org/advice/ask/2005/10/31/bicycling2/index.html
http://www.treehugger.com/files/2005/10/confirmed_air_q.php

Hiking
http://www.americanhiking.org/events/ntd/faq.html
http://www.britannica.com/eb/article-9019830/Camp-David

Swimming
http://ezinearticles.com/?Saline-versus-Chlorine---Which-is-Best-For-Your-Hot-Tub-or-
    Pool?&id=195836
http://www.bccresearch.com/chm/sampleCHM032B.pdf

IN FRONT OF THE MIRROR AND IN THE BATHROOM
Baby Oil
http://www.care2.com/channels/solutions/self/499
http://www.edelweissbotanicals.com/faq.htm
http://www.uoregon.edu/~recycle/TRIVIA.htm
http://www.usatoday.com/news/health/2006-11-21-births_x.htm
http://ntp-server.niehs.nih.gov/ntp/roc/eleventh/profiles/s114mine.pdf
http://auto.howstuffworks.com/question417.htm

Bath Salts/Bubble Bath
http://www.epa.gov/performancetrack/tools/wasteman.htm
http://www.amazon.com/Sesame-Street-Bubble-Berry-Burst/dp/B00005303J/
    ref=pd_sim_hpc_3/104-3264657-7247119?ie=UTF8
http://www.mcelwee.net/html/densities_of_various_materials.html
http://www.ballparks.com/baseball/national/wrigle.htm

Conditioner
http://www.nclnet.org/general/Package%20report/nclreport.htm

Cotton Balls
http://www.autexrj.org/No1/old1_2.pdf

Deodorant
http://www.thegreenguide.com/reports/product.mhtml?id=43&sec=3
http://en.wikipedia.org/wiki/Aluminum
http://www.hardman.com.au/Antiperspirant%20Actives.htm
http://www.ratebeer.com/Story.asp?StoryID=385
http://www.mid.org/services/save/hm-appl-cost-2006.htm

Eyeliner
http://www.lesstoxicguide.ca/print.asp?mode=whole#eyeli
http://www.packagedfacts.com/product/print/default.asp?productid=328914
http://www.google.com/search?num=50&hl=en&lr=&q=eyeliner+pencil+weighs+grams

Eye Shadow
http://bizrate.lycos.com/cosmetics/eye_makeup--eye_shadow/products_att259818--97200-4127_att290519--271598-_show--120.html
http://findarticles.com/p/articles/mi_m4021/is_n3_v19/ai_19165299/pg_2

Foundation
http://www.sks-bottle.com/preadd.php4?01380010.02S&2511-19&2511-19B
http://www.energy.ca.gov

Hair Dye
http://www.thegreenguide.com/doc.mhtml?i=110&s=hair
http://www.livingnaturally.com/PDFDocs/u/UW6XK1WH83KS8KCKCN5905XVXSSKAL98.PDF
http://www.lesstoxicguide.ca/print.asp?mode=whole#hairc

Lipstick
http://www.lesstoxicguide.ca/print.asp?mode=whole#found
http://www.thegreenguide.com/reports/product.mhtml?id=42&sec=3
http://www.packagedfacts.com/product/print/default.asp?productid=328914

Lotions
http://www.sks-bottle.com/340c/fin78.html
http://www.csun.edu/science/BFl/waste_stats.html
http://www.staytan.com/bothuyfree.php

Mascara
http://www.ewg.org/news/story.php?id=4964
http://www.lesstoxicguide.ca/print.asp?mode=whole#masca

http://www.ashlandfood.coop/pdf/packaging%20study.pdf
http://www.eia.doe.gov/kids/energyfacts/saving/recycling/solidwaste/sourcereduction.html

Perfume/Cologne
http://www.checnet.org/healthehouse/education/articles-detail.asp?Main_ID=509
http://www.alive.com/793a2a2.php?subject_bread_cramb=75
http://www.phthalates.org/whatare/index.asp
http://en.wikipedia.org/wiki/Phthalates
http://www.phthalates.com/index.asp?page=54

Shampoo
http://www.p2pays.org/ref/20/19893.htm
http://www.mid.org/services/save/hm-appl-cost-2006.htm
http://www.eia.doe.gov/emeu/reps/enduse/er01_us_tab1.html
http://www.nclnet.org/general/Package%20report/nclreport.htm

Shaving Gel/Foam
http://www.greenchoices.org/toiletries.html
http://www.madehow.com/Volume-1/Shaving-Cream.html
http://www.cfsan.fda.gov/~dms/cos-lab3.html
http://www.spe.org/spe/jsp/basic/0,,1104_1732,00.html
http://www.eia.doe.gov/emeu/steo/pub/special/mtbecost.html
http://www.mid.org/services/save/hm-appl-cost-2006.htm

Soap
http://www.womenshealthcaretopics.com/bn_bathshower_Shower_Gels_Body_Washes.
    htm
http://www.kirksnatural.com/faqs.html

Sponges
http://www.womenshealthcaretopics.com/bn_bathshower_Various_Bath_and_
    Shower_Aids.htm
http://www.nrdc.org/water/drinking/uscities/pdf/chap05.pdf

Tampons
http://www.lesstoxicguide.ca/print.asp?mode=whole
http://www.pbs.org/pov/borders/2004/talk/uf_170.html
http://www.seac.org/tampons/environment.shtml
http://www.ehponline.org/members/2002/110p23-28devito/tab3.gif
http://www.femininehygiene.com/organic_cotton_tampons.htm

The Big Picture

http://www.findarticles.com/p/articles/mi_m1571/is_n25_v14/ai_20884032
http://www.biz.uiowa.edu/bizfolio/2005/katelynquinn/Athletic%20Footwear%20
    Industry.doc

http://www.pubmedcentral.nih.gov/articlerender.fcgi?artid=1459948
http://www.worldwatch.org/pubs/mag/204/172/mos
http://en.wikipedia.org/wiki/Over-illumination
http://www.lighting4sport.com/lightpollution.htm
http://www.earthscan.co.uk/news/article/mps/uan/713/v/5/sp/
http://www.ehponline.org/members/2006/114-5/focus.html
http://english.people.com.cn/200506/15/eng20050615_190415.html

The Simple Steps

RENT
http://www.answers.com/topic/alps
http://money.cnn.com/magazines/fortune/fortune_archive/2005/05/30/8261249/index.htm
http://www.thegreenguide.org/article/recreation/sports

FOOTWEAR
http://www.cwc.org/tires/97-1rpt.pdf
http://www.notoxicburning.org/recycling.html
http://www.oberlin.edu/recycle/facts.html
http://www.drpribut.com/sports/sneaker_odyssey.html
http://basketball.ballparks.com/NBA/IndianaPacers/newindex.htm

LITTER
http://cbs.sportsline.com/general/story/8552075
http://sunnyvale.ca.gov/Departments/Public+Works/Solid+Waste+and+Recycling/
    Residential+Services/SingleFamily/Cloth+Diaper+Information.htm

The Little Things

EQUIPMENT
Bags
http://www.earthpak.com/grandeduffledufflesports-cpmazma.html
http://www.usnwc.org/involved_sponsorship.asp
http://www.americanplasticscouncil.org/s_apc/sec.asp?CID=312&DID=930

Balls
http://www.jumpusa.com/tennis_equipment.html
http://www0.shopping.com/xPC-Lob_Ster_Tretorn_Prolite_Pressureless_Tennis_Balls_
    Pack_of_90
http://www.itftennis.com/technical/questions/
http://www.usopen.org/en_US/about/index.html
http://www.mapcrow.info/Distance_between_London_UK_and_New_York_US.html

Bats
http://www.secat.net/docs/resources/US_Energy_Requirements_for_Aluminum_Production.
    pdf
http://www.slambats.com/about.asp#Why_Hit_with_Wood
http://www.hitrunscore.com/baseball-bats-buyers-guide.html#anchor14

http://www.hitrunscore.com/baseball-bats-buyers-guide.html
http://www.p2pays.org/ref/08/07530.pdf
http://www.littleleague.org/MEDIA/2006jamboreecloses.asp
http://www.bts.gov/publications/national_transportation_statistics/html/table_04_21.html
http://www.littleleague.org/media/2006llbbseriesinfo.asp

Bicycles

http://www.mctselect.com/cgi-bin/krt/download/20060626-BIKEFRAME.pdf?doc=
    KRT%2Fkrtonepages%2Fdocs%2F002%2F456&filetype=wmark_pdf
http://www.geocities.com/sirflakeyjake/GGsustain.html
http://strongframes.com/material_tech/metallurgy/3/
http://deq.state.ms.us/Mdeq.nsf/page/Recycling_RecyclingTrivia?OpenDocument
http://www.minesandcommunities.org/Action/press1046.pdf
http://www.wrenchscience.com/WSLogic/Frames.aspx?material=steel&styleCode=R
http://www.cicle.org/news/hotcakes.html

Donate

http://www.thegreenguide.org/article/recreation/sports
http://www.goodwillswfl.org/RetailDonations/estimate_value.htm
http://www.ngf.org/cgi/whofaqa.asp
http://turf.lib.msu.edu/2000s/2000/000106.pdf
http://www.onlygolfballs.com/cat25_1.htm

Equipment—General

http://www.g-forse.com/enviro/actionsport.html
http://www.pubmedcentral.nih.gov/articlerender.fcgi?artid=1459948
http://www.udel.edu/PR/UDaily/2005/mar/rwool080405.html
http://www.explainthatstuff.com/composites.html

Equipment—Used

http://articles.moneycentral.msn.com/SavingandDebt/FindDealsOnline/10thingsYou
    ShouldntBuyNew.aspx
http://www.nsga.org/public/pages/index.cfm?pageid=1435
http://www.nsga.org/public/pages/index.cfm?pageid=1436

Gloves and Mitts

http://www.osti.gov/bridge/servlets/purl/10134188-BBjWAH/native/10134188.pdf
http://www.littleleague.org/MEDIA/2006jamboreecloses.asp
http://members.tripod.com/bb_catchers/catchers/equip1.htm

Golf Clubs

http://www.opalent.com/Facts/index.php
http://www.evergreenfire.net/
http://findarticles.com/p/articles/mi_qa4031/is_200306/ai_n9276392
http://www.indiana.edu/~nca/monographs/10golf.shtml
http://www.worldgolf.com/wglibrary/articles/equipguide.html
http://www.ga.wa.gov/visitor/facts.htm

Helmets

http://www.helmets.org/recycle.htm
http://www.aappublications.org/cgi/content/full/pediatrics;108/4/1030
http://faculty.washington.edu/chudler/bikelaw.html
http://bicycling.about.com/od/helmets/a/helmetbasics.htm
http://www.helmets.org/sizing.htm
http://www.nascar.com/races/tracks/bms/index.html#null

Surfboards

http://www.surfrider.org/a-z/surfboards.asp
http://www.thegreenguide.com/doc.mhtml?i=116&s=surfboards
http://www.alternative-hawaii.com/oahu1.htm

Tennis Rackets

http://www.plasticsmakeitpossible.org/s_microsite/sec_athletics.asp?CID=489&DID=1466
http://www.tenniscompany.com/ABOUT6.html
http://www.tennis.com/yourgame/gear/racquets/tecnifibre/tecnifibre.aspx?id=873
http://www.americansportsdata.com/pr-participantsportmethodology.asp
http://www.e4s.org.uk/textilesonline/content/6library/report4/5_knitted_nylon.htm

Water Bottles

http://cbs.sportsline.com/general/story/8552075

Yoga Mats

http://www.yesmagazine.org/article.asp?ID=1433
http://www.yogamatters.com/acatalog/Trade_secrets_2.html
http://abcnews.go.com/Health/WomensHealth/story?id=2243106&page=1
http://www.extremescience.com/HighestElevation.htm

PLAYING AND PARTICIPATING

Baseball/Softball

http://www.seattle.gov/parks/parkspaces/JeffersonPark/documents/deis.pdf
http://www.mid.org/services/save/hm-appl-cost-2006.htm
http://www.safeusa.org/sports/baseball.htm
http://www.ci.durham.nc.us/departments/parks/fees.cfm#11

Basketball

http://www.advancedbuildings.net/documents/gymnasium.pdf
http://www.nike.com/nikebiz/nikebiz.jhtml;bsessionid=Z3E435S4324QACQFTBFCF5AKA
    WMB2IZB?page=27&cat=nikegoplaces
http://www.nike.com/nikebiz/nikebiz.jhtml?page=27&cat=reuseashoe&subcat=us-surface
http://upcoming.org/event/71429/

Cycling

http://www.congress.gov/cgi-bin/cpquery/R?cp109:FLD010:@1(hr570)
http://www.amazon.com/exec/obidos/ASIN/B000A8NQQC/dealtime-sg-ret-20/ref=nosim

http://www.epa.gov/epaoswer/non-hw/green/pubs/rubber.pdf
http://www.iht.com/articles/ap/2006/10/26/sports/EU_SPT_CYC_Tour_de_France_Route_
    Glance.php

Football and Soccer
http://www.turfgrassod.org/lawninstitute/environmental_benefits.htm
http://en.wikipedia.org/wiki/Artificial_turf
http://new.turfgrasssod.org/pdfs/Recorded_Temperature_Comparisons_Chart.pdf
http://www.turfgrassod.org/webarticles/anmviewer.asp?a=130&z=37
http://www.turfgrassod.org/webarticles/anmviewer.asp?a=131&z=36

Golf
http://www.golfandenvironment.org/ecofriendlygolf.htm
http://www.earthsmartconsumer.com/golf.html
http://www.auduboninternational.org/projects/mlp/envioutcomesgolf.htm
http://www.livescience.com/othernews/050909_golf_pesticides.html
http://www.masters.org/en_US/info/faq/index.html

Hockey
http://ctec-varennes.rncan.gc.ca/fichier.php/codectec/En/2003-066-6/2003-066-6f.pdf
http://www.mid.org/services/save/hm-appl-cost-2006.htm
http://www.arlingtonva.us/Departments/CountyManager/Documents/8047ice%20
    rink%20fact%20sheet%2010-06.doc
https://oss.ticketmaster.com/html/pack_searchtix.html?1=EN&CNTX=453074

Skiing/Snowboarding
http://www.pubmedcentral.nih.gov/articlerender.fcgi?artid=1459948
http://www.timewarner.com/corp/newsroom/pr/0,20812,153257,00.html
http://www.nsaa.org/nsaa/press/facts-ski-snbd-safety.asp

Surfing
http://www.ecosurfproject.org/resources/articles/ecosurferextra/index.php?sectID=beach
http://www.npr.org/programs/morning/features/patc/surfboard/
http://www.wrcc.dri.edu/narratives/CALIFORNIA.htm

Tennis
http://www.eere.energy.gov/buildings/database/energy.cfm?ProjectID=282
http://blogs.business2.com/waterlog/2007/01/1st_tidal_power.html

The Big Picture

http://news.moneycentral.msn.com/ticker/article.asp?Feed=BW&Date=20060912&ID=601
    3253&Symbol=US:HIT
http://www.deluxe.com
http://www.federalreserve.gov/boardDocs/press/other/2004/20041206/default.htm

http://www.nacha.org/news/default.htm
http://www.consumercredit.com/
http://www.csmonitor.com/2006/0110/dailyUpdate.html
http://www.ens-newswire.com/ens/sep2002/2002-09-09-01.asp

The Simple Steps

ATM RECEIPTS
http://news.moneycentral.msn.com/ticker/article.asp?Feed=BW&Date=20060912&
    ID=6013253&Symbol=US:HIT

AUTOMATIC DEPOSIT
http://nacha.org/OtherResources/Direct_Deposit_and_Direct_Payment_General_
    Information_-_2nd_Edition.pdf

PAPERLESS BANK STATEMENTS
http://www.clickz.com/showPage.html?page=746351
http://www.collegeboard.com/student/pay/add-it-up/4494.html

The Little Things

Advisers
http://www.pueblo.gsa.gov/cic_text/money/stockbroker/broker.htm
http://www.socialinvestmentforum.org/areas/research/trends/sri_trends_report_2005.pdf

Brokerage Statements
http://www.nyse.com/about/history/1022743347410.html

Checks
http://www.deluxe.com
http://www.federalreserve.gov/boardDocs/press/other/2004/20041206/default.htm
http://www.house.gov/rothman/ontheissues/iraqwarcosts.htm

Electronic Payments
http://www.nacha.org/news/default.htm
http://ask.yahoo.com/20040209.html
http://www.consumercredit.com/

Electronic Tax Refunds
http://www.irs.gov/newsroom/article/0,,id=152048,00.html
http://www.msnbc.msn.com/id/7069656
http://www.occ.treas.gov/netbank/FurstandNolleACHPolicyPaper6.pdf
http://www.ocgov.com/press/pdf/september.pdf

Online Banking
http://www.bai.org/BANKINGSTRATEGIES/2006-sep-oct/PaymentsStrategies/cashdebit/
    print.asp

Paperless Accounting
http://www.bizjournals.com/triad/stories/2006/09/11/focus1.html?b=1157947200%5E13
  42250
http://www.clui.org/clui_4_1/lotl/v23/v23c.html

Prospectuses
http://www.forbes.com/lists/2006/54/biz_06rich400_The-400-Richest-Americans_Rank_
  15.html
http://www.xerox.com/Static_HTML/xsis/autmfulf.htm
https://ics.adp.com/release11/public_site/products/invco/intelprint.html

Proxy Statements
https://ics.adp.com/release11/public_site/about/stats.html
http://www.casavaria.com/eco/epi/020917air.htm
http://www.opensecrets.org/news/accountants/index.asp

Socially Responsible Investing
http://www.csmonitor.com/2006/0110/dailyUpdate.html
http://www.innovestgroup.com/index.php?option=com_content&task=view&id=34&
  Itemid=32
http://www.socialinvestmentforum.org/areas/research/trends/sri_trends_report_2005.pdf
http://www.ens-newswire.com/ens/sep2002/2002-09-09-01.asp

Stock Certificates
http://www.sia.com/stp/pdf/PhysCertGuide2alternatives.pdf

Tax Forms
http://links.jstor.org/sici?sici=0002-9092(197311)55%3A4%3C633%3ALPIAH%
  3E2.0.CO%3B2-R
http://www.urbanext.uiuc.edu/apples/facts.html
http://www.rainforest-alliance.org/aar.cfm?id=conservation
http://www2.sims.berkeley.edu/research/projects/how-much-info-2003/print.htm
http://www.irs.gov/pub/irs-pdf/f1040.pdf
http://www.irs.gov/newsroom/article/0,,id=152048,00.html
http://www.irs.gov/efile/article/0,,id=118508,00.html
http://www.findarticles.com/p/articles/mi_m2893/is_3_25/ai_n16361291

Trade Confirmations
http://www.millenniumcampaign.org/site/pp.asp?c=grKVL2NLE&b=185518
http://www.borgenproject.org
http://www.world-exchanges.org

Withdrawals/Deposits
http://money.cnn.com/magazines/fortune/fortune_archive/2004/07/26/377172/index.htm
http://findarticles.com/p/articles/mi_qa3678/is_199707/ai_n8775215
http://www.federalreserve.gov/boardDocs/press/other/2004/20041206/default.htm
http://www.usfst.com/pastissue/article.asp?art=26906&issue=166

11

The Big Picture

http://www.holistichealthtools.com/air_quality.html
http://go.ucsusa.org/publications/nucleus.cfm?publicationID=242
http://www.rcgov.org/pubworks/water/facts_about_water_use.pdf
http://www.countryenergy.com.au/internet/cewebpub.nsf/AttachmentsByTitle/
    flib-energyeff/$file/es_windows.pdf
http://www.worldwatch.org/
http://www.energymatch.com/features/article.asp?articleid=4
http://www.insulate.org/consumerinfo.html#2
http://www.earthshare.org/tips/00-fall.txt
http://www.wikipedia.org/wiki/Energy_conservation
http://www.nah
http://www.hgtv.com/hgtv/rm_home_building_other/article/0,1797,HGTV_3727_352976
    1,00.html
http://peakstoprairies.org/topichub/PrintPage.cfm?hub=31&subsec=13&nav=1
http://www.bentonvillear.com/docs/bldg/erosion_control_home_builders.pdf

The Simple Steps

ENERGY STAR
http://www.energystar.gov/index.cfm?c=news.nr_news

LOW-FLOW PLUMBING
http://www.epa.gov/water/you/intro.html

CEILING FANS
http://go.ucsusa.org/publications/nucleus.cfm?publicationID=242

The Little Things

Absorbent Materials
http://seattlepi.nwsource.com/specials/brokenpromises/288235_stormwatersolutions11.asp
http://www.metrokc.gov/dnrp/swd/greenbuilding/documents/Green_home_
    remodel-landscaping.pdf
http://www.co.ramsey.mn.us/NR/rdonlyres/2ACE0C58-C5E7-4C98-B182-37103BD69C9E/
    3753/StopWaterPamphlet061.pdf

Adhesives
http://www.aiacolorado.org/SDRG/div09/index.html
http://www.greenbuilder.com/sourcebook/FinishesAdhesives.html#ADHESIVES
http://oikos.com/news/2004/08.html
http://www.electric.austin.tx.us/energy%20efficiency/programs/green%20building/
    Sourcebook/constructionAdhesives.htm

Air-Conditioning
http://www.energystar.gov/ia/new_homes/features/EstarAirConditioners1-17-01.pdf
http://www.slate.com/id/2147167/nav/tap1/

http://www.voanews.com/english/archive/2005-09/Bush-Clinton-Katrina-Fund-Raises-96-
    Million-Dollars.cfm

Bathroom Countertops
http://www.greenhomeguide.com/index.php/product_detail/414/C166
http://www.rv.org/EB-16455.htm
http://www.homeenergy.org/archive/hem.dis.anl.gov/eehem/95/951110.html
http://www.homedepot.com/pre180/HDUS/EN_US/diy_main/pg_diy.jsp?prod_id=1004142
    59&cm_mmc=1hd.com2froogle-_-product_feed-_-D29X-_-100414259

Carpet
http://www.grist.org/news/daily/2004/12/01/5/index.html
http://www.coloryourcarpet.com/Environment/Landfillstats2.html

Cooling/Heating Systems
http://www.drivecleanacrosstexas.org/for_teachers/grades_9-12/unit1/lesson2.stm
http://www.riverdeep.net/current/2002/03/032502t_cowpower.jhtml
http://www.energystar.gov/ia/products/heat_cool/GUIDE_2COLOR.pdf
http://www.energystar.gov/index.cfm?c=heat_cool.pr_hvac

Create an Envelope
http://www.nbm.org/Exhibits/greenHouse2/principles/principles.html
http://www.theicct.org/documents/RichardFraer-1.pdf

Drywall
http://www.ecoact.org/Programs/Green_Building/green_Materials/gypsum.htm
http://www.pulverdryerusa.com/applications.html#wallboard
http://en.wikipedia.org/wiki/Great_Wall_of_China

Dual-Flush Toilets
http://www.treehugger.com/files/2005/03/dual_flush_toil_1.php
http://en.wikipedia.org/wiki/Sports_league_attendances
http://sjr.state.fl.us/programs/outreach/pubs/order/pdfs/as_survey.pdf
http://factfinder.census.gov/servlet/STTable?_bm=y&-geo_id=01000US&-qr_name=ACS_
    2005_EST_G00_S2504&-ds_name=ACS_2005_EST_G00
http://www.epa.gov/OW/you/chap3.html

Erosion/Sedimentation
http://www.builtgreen.net/faqs.html
http://www.des.state.nh.us/factsheets/sp/sp-1.htm
http://muextension.missouri.edu/explore/agguides/agengin/g01509.htm
http://www.deq.state.mi.us/documents/deq-land-sesc-manualunit1.pdf
http://www.pasadena.com/rose_bowl.asp

Fabrics
http://www.terratex.com/launch.html
http://www.decoratorsupplyinc.com/yardage.htm

http://www.terratex.com/pdf/terratext2.pdf
http://www.answers.com/topic/broadwoven-fabric-mills-manmade-fiber-and-silk
http://www.greatbrook.com/E135/Waterbeds_East.pdf
http://www.mid.org/services/save/hm-appl-cost-2006.htm
http://quickfacts.census.gov/qfd/states/36000.html

Finishes
http://www.homeenergy.org/archive/hem.dis.anl.gov/eehem/94/940509.html
http://www.eia.doe.gov/emeu/reps/enduse/er01_us_tab1.html
http://www.energystar.gov/index.cfm?c=roof_prods.pr_roof_products
http://www.energystar.gov/index.cfm?c=roof_prods.pr_roof_faqs
http://www.energy.ca.gov/2005publications/CEC-300-2005-013/CEC-300-2005-013-FS.PDF
http://pentagon.afis.osd.mil/facts-area.cfm

Furniture
http://www.worldwatch.org/node/1490
http://www.sierraclub.org/sierra/200511/tr1.asp
http://www.eia.doe.gov/oiaf/servicerpt/cafe/cafe_tbls.html
http://www.rainforestfoundation.org/library.php
http://quickfacts.census.gov/qfd/states/01000.html

Garage
http://www.house-n-home-building.com/newsletters/house-building-january05.htm
http://www.e-star.com/publications/andrews/garage_to_house_issue.pdf
http://www.globalgreen.org/gbrc/whygreen.htm

Glass Tiles
http://www.ecowise.com/green/tile/gtile.shtml
http://www.mid.org/services/save/hm-appl-cost-2006.htm
http://www.osti.gov/bridge/servlets/purl/816041-pzriki/webviewable/816041.pdf
http://www.repp.org/geothermal/geothermal_brief_power_technologyandgeneration.html

Greenfields vs. Brownfields
http://www.aspencore.org/sitepages/pid94.php
http://www.builditgreen.org/newconstructionguidelines.pdf
http://www.housingandenvironment.org/Text%20Files/brownfieldsfinal.pdf
http://www.fs.fed.us/projects/four-threats/
http://www.brownfieldscenter.org/small/faq.shtml
http://quickfacts.census.gov/qfd/states/25000.html

Hardwood Flooring
http://www.thegreenguide.com/reports/product.mhtml?id=70&sec=3
http://www.builditgreen.org/resource/index.cfm?fuseaction=factsheet_detail&rowid=4
http://www.neo.state.ne.us/home_const/factsheets/min_use_lumber.htm
http://www.chickasawflooring.com/flooringestimator.shtml
http://www.carbohydrateeconomy.org/library/admin/uploadedfiles/Cooperative_Forestry_
    Takes_Root.htm

http://www.ams.usda.gov/tmd/FSMIP/FY2004/IN0421mktrpt.pdf
http://www.fs.fed.us/ne/warren/long.html
http://www.nlc.org/about_cities/cities_101/138.cfm

Highly Reflective Roofing

http://www.homeenergy.org/archive/hem.dis.anl.gov/eehem/94/940509.html
http://www.eia.doe.gov/emeu/reps/enduse/er01_us_tab1.html
http://www.energystar.gov/index.cfm?c=roof_prods.pr_roof_products
http://www.energystar.gov/index.cfm?c=roof_prods.pr_roof_faqs
http://www.energy.ca.gov/2005publications/CEC-300-2005-013/CEC-300-2005-013-
    FS.PDF
http://pentagon.afis.osd.mil/facts-area.cfm

Insulation

http://www.applegateinsulation.com/environmental.aspx#
http://www.epa.gov/epaoswer/osw/specials/funfacts/maintence.htm
http://www.thegreenguide.com/doc.mhtml?i=ask&s=insulation
http://www.census.gov/const/newressales.xls
http://www.eia.doe.gov/emeu/reps/enduse/er01_us_tab1.html
http://quickfacts.census.gov/qfd/states/34/3474000.html

Insulated Wall Panels

http://www.austinenergy.com/Energy%20Efficiency/Programs/Green%20Building/
    Resources/Fact%20Sheets/ICFs.pdf
http://www.sips.org/DesktopModules/Pictures/PictureView.aspx?tabID=0&ItemID=1321&
    mid=14127&wversion=Staging
http://www.sips.org/portal/tabid_5768/Default.aspx
http://www.eia.doe.gov/emeu/reps/enduse/er01_us_tab1.html
http://www.eia.doe.gov/kids/energyfacts/science/energy_calculator.html
http://www.lewrockwell.com/reisman/reisman15.html

Kitchen Countertops

http://www.grist.org/advice/ask/2006/07/24/countertops/index.html
http://amicusgreen.com/v1/PaperStone%20Certified%20Brochure.pdf
http://amicusgreen.com/v1/Ecoverings-cutsheet.pdf
http://www.marketresearch.com/product/display.asp?productid=1187213&g=1
http://www.theoceans.net/expguide/navigation.htm

Landscaping

http://www.epa.gov/greenacres/nativeplants/factsht.html
http://www.uvm.edu/pss/ppp/articles/fuels.html

Lighting

http://www.energystar.gov/index.cfm?c=cfls.pr_cfls
http://www.renewables.com
http://www.ciwmb.ca.gov/GreenBuilding/Basics.htm

Linoleum vs. Vinyl

http://www.grist.org/advice/ask/2006/02/06/flooring/index.html
http://www.thegreenguide.com/doc.mhtml?i=96&s=eco-renovation
http://www.thegreenguide.com/doc.mhtml?i=ask&s=flooring
http://www.naturalhomerugs.com/vinyl-tiles.php
http://www.ecologycenter.org/ptf/report1996/report1996_01.html
http://press.arrivenet.com/industry/article.php/690349.html
http://www.washingtonpost.com/wp-srv/liveonline/03/special/nation/sp_iraq_felmy
031403.htm

Natural Site Features

http://www.nipc.org/environment/sustainable/development/communities/BSC%20
Series%20Sustainable%20Sites%20and%20Natural%20Landscapes.pdf
http://competition.globalgreen.org/green_building/05_twenty_strats_1.php
http://www.lowimpactdevelopment.org/lid%20articles/seattledjc_jul25_2002.pdf

Orientation

http://www.austinenergy.com/Energy%20Efficiency/Programs/Green%20Building/
Resources/Fact%20Sheets/easyGreenIdeas.pdf
http://www.fsec.ucf.edu/BLDG/fyh/priority/index.htm

Paint

http://www.productstewardship.us/supportingdocs/DialoguePaintPS.doc#_Toc67675253
http://www.p2pays.org/ref/26/25292/25292.pdf
http://www.p2pays.org/ref/26/25292/curriculum_spreadsheets_manual.xls
http://www.gsa.gov/Portal/gsa/ep/contentView.do?pageTypeId=8199&channelId=-
13259&P=XI&contentId=9022&contentType=GSA_BASIC
http://www.seattle.gov/dpd/stellent/groups/pan/@pan/@sustainableblding/documents/
web_informational/dpds_007583.pdf
http://www.lao.ca.gov/2000/051100_cal_travels/051100_cal_travels_intro.html
http://ceres.ca.gov/ceres/calweb/40tips.html

Porous Pavement

http://www.stormwatercenter.net/Assorted%20Fact%20Sheets/Tool6_Stormwater_Practic
es/Infiltration%20Practice/
http://en.wikipedia.org/wiki/Permeable_paving
http://en.wikipedia.org/wiki/Asphalt
http://www.landdevelopmenttoday.com/index.php?name=News&file=article&sid=632&
theme=Printer
http://www.bdcnetwork.com/article/CA6297622.html

Roof

http://en.wikipedia.org/wiki/Green_roof
http://www.epa.gov/heatislands/strategies/coolroofs.html

Shade

http://www.alliantenergy.com/docs/groups/public/documents/pub/p015121.hcsp
http://www.rockdale.nsw.gov.au/cms/cmswebcontent.nsf/Content/Environment_
    Cando_Energy_Home
http://www.austinenergy.com/energy%20efficiency/programs/Green%20Building/
    Sourcebook/energySavingLandscapes.htm
http://www.eia.doe.gov/emeu/reps/enduse/er01_us_tab1.html
http://www.census.gov/Press-Release/www/releases/archives/census_2000/001113.html
http://www.webflyer.com/travel/milemarker/getmileage.php?city=PHX&city=MIA&
    city=&city=&city=&bonus=0&bonus_use_min=0&class_bonus=0&class_bonus_
    use_min=0&promo_bonus=0&promo_bonus_use_min=0&min=0&min_type=
    m&ticket_price=
http://www.bts.gov/publications/national_transportation_statistics/html/table_04_21.html
http://quickfacts.census.gov/qfd/states/04/0455000.html

Site Selection

http://www.greenbuilder.com/general/articles/AAS.SiteSelection.html
http://www.usatourist.com/english/tips/maps.html#map

Slopes

http://www.greenbuilder.com/general/articles/AAS.SiteSelection.html
http://www.builditgreen.org/newconstructionguidelines.pdf
http://www.recycleworks.org/greenbuilding/sus_sitework.html

Soil

http://www.builtgreen.net/faqs.html
http://www.ecocycle.org/pdfs/Eco-facts_2004.pdf
http://www.diynetwork.com/diy/home_building/article/0,2085,DIY_13953_2512187,00.html
http://www.green.ca.gov/EPP/Grounds/mulch.htm
http://www.greenguardian.com/eppg/9_1.asp

Solar

http://www.solcomhouse.com/solarpower.htm

Solar Water Heaters

http://www.solardirect.com/swh/swh.htm
http://www.ases.org/aboutre/faq.htm
http://www.epa.gov/water/you/chap1.html

Treated Wood

http://www.moea.state.mn.us/publications/hhw-treatedwood.pdf
http://greenguardian.com/EPPG/8_1.asp
http://www.lycos.com/info/decking.html
http://www.sciencenews.org/articles/20040131/bob9.asp
http://www.chickasawflooring.com/flooringestimator.shtm
http://www.austinwholesaledecking.com/redwood.htm

Trees

http://www.landscape-america.com/landscapes/design/design.html
http://www.fs.fed.us/psw/programs/cufr/research/studies_detail.php?ProjID=59
http://www.eia.doe.gov/emeu/reps/enduse/er01_us_tab1.html
http://www.ucsusa.org/clean_energy/fossil_fuels/offmen-how-coal-works.html

Windbreaks

http://www.austinenergy.com/energy%20efficiency/programs/Green%20Building/
    Sourcebook/energySavingLandscapes.htm
http://www.epa.gov/reg3esd1/garden/heat.htm
http://ianrpubs.unl.edu/forestry/ec1772.htm
http://www.eia.doe.gov/emeu/reps/enduse/er01_us_tab1.html
http://www.ers.usda.gov/StateFacts/US.HTM
http://www.akenergyauthority.org/AEAdocuments/REPV1ExecutiveSummary.pdf

Windows

http://www.energystar.gov/index.cfm?c=windows_doors.pr_savemoney#1
http://buildingsdatabook.eren.doe.gov/docs/2.1.7.pdf
http://buildingsdatabook.eren.doe.gov/docs/5.5.1.pdf

Wood

http://www.thegreenguide.com/doc.mhtml?i=108&s=wood
http://www.nps.gov/archive/yose/nature/nature.htm
http://www.nrdc.org/land/forests/qcert.asp#2

The Simple Steps

http://www.epa.gov
http://www.nativeenergy.com

The Little Things

http://www.epa.gov
http://www.nativeenergy.com

index of tips

acknowledgments

The Green Book could not have been possible without Colleen Howell, PhD, whose research and writing helped pull it all together. We thank you. Cameron Diaz and William McDonough helped create this book before it was even a book. A special thanks to them. Susan Raihofer has been a gift of support and guidance. Skye Hoppus was instrumental to this book happening. We'd also like to thank each of our contributors for their time, their attention, and, of course, their personal, hilarious, thoughtful, and insightful anecdotes: Ellen DeGeneres, Robert Redford, Will Ferrell, Jennifer Aniston, Tim McGraw, Faith Hill, Martha Stewart, Tyra Banks, Dale Earnhardt Jr., Tiki Barber, Owen Wilson, and Justin Timberlake. And for their support, friendship, guidance, counsel, and patience, thanks to Andrew Beebe, Peter Berg, Mary Choteborsky, Billy Connelly, Julie Darmody, Joyce Deep, Keith Estabrook, Stanley Fields, Tierney Gearon, Jade Gurss, James Joaquin, Zem Joaquin, Debbie Levin, Mark Lepselter, Matti Leshem, Jesse Lutz, Carolyn McGuinness, Linda Meltzer, Gaby Morgerman, Michael Muller, Elise Peach, Margaret Sanders, Jennifer Sbranti, Liana Schwarz, Ina Treciokas, Elana Weiss, Rachael Yarbrough, Julie Yorn, and Kevin Yorn.

about the authors

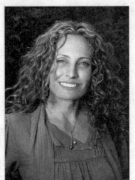

Michael Muller

Elizabeth Rogers has worked with the Natural Resources Defense Council, and she has created and produced MTV's eco-friendly show *Trippin*. She is currently an environmental consultant and lives with her son in Venice, California. She tries to shift a habit daily.

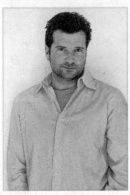

Tierney Gearon

Thomas M. Kostigen writes the "Ethics Monitor" column for *Dow Jones MarketWatch*. A longtime journalist and former Bloomberg News editor, he has written works that have appeared in numerous publications around the world.

about this book

A portion of the proceeds from the sales of **The Green Book** is being put toward the Green Book Foundation to support environmental causes and nonprofit organizations.

The Green Book is printed using 100 percent postconsumer recycled paper.

For the interior, using 100 percent postconsumer recycled paper instead of virgin fiber paper reduces our ecological footprint by the following amounts for every ton of paper:
trees: 17
solid waste: 1,080 pounds
water: 10,196 gallons
suspended particles in the water: 6.8 pounds
air emissions: 2,372 pounds

One ton of paper is used to print four thousand copies of **The Green Book**.

The cover stock is also made of 100 percent postconsumer recycled fiber, which means:
No New Trees → Neutral pH → Totally Chlorine Free → Archival → Acid Free

The Green Book's production energy has been carbon offset by Native Energy: *www.nativeenergy.com.*

For additional information and resources, visit:
www.readthegreenbook.com.